BACK ON TRACK

BACK ON TRACK

• • • • • • •

A PRACTICAL GUIDE TO HELP
KIDS OF ALL AGES THRIVE

Dr. Rebecca Jackson

Mayo Clinic Press

MAYO CLINIC PRESS
200 First St. SW
Rochester, MN 55905
mcpress.mayoclinic.org

The information in this book is true and complete to the best of our knowledge. This book is
intended as an informative guide for those wishing to learn more about health issues. It is not
intended to replace, countermand or conflict with advice given to you by your own physician.
The ultimate decision concerning your care should be made between you and your doctor.
Information in this book is offered with no guarantees. The author and publisher disclaim all
liability in connection with the use of this book.

The views expressed are the author's personal views, and do not necessarily reflect the policy or
position of Mayo Clinic.

To stay informed about Mayo Clinic Press, please subscribe to our free e-newsletter at
mcpress.mayoclinic.org or follow us on social media.

For bulk sales to employers, member groups and health-related companies, contact Mayo
Clinic at SpecialSalesMayoBooks@mayo.edu.

Proceeds from the sale of every book benefit important medical research and education at
Mayo Clinic.

Cover design by D. Soleil Paz
Cover art: Heads © CHUENMANUSE/SHUTTERSTOCK.COM; Scribble lines © FROGELLA/
SHUTTERSTOCK.COM

Library of Congress Cataloging-in-Publication Data

Names: Jackson, Rebecca, (Cognitive specialist), author.
Title: Back on track : a practical guide to help kids of all ages thrive / by Rebecca Jackson.
Description: First edition. | Rochester, MN : Mayo Clinic Press, 2023. | Includes
    bibliographical references. |
Identifiers: LCCN 2023009374 (print) | LCCN 2023009375 (ebook) | ISBN
    9798887700618 (paperback) | ISBN 9798887700625 (epub)
Subjects: LCSH: Child development. | Child psychology. | COVID-19 Pandemic, 2020—
    Psychological aspects.
Classification: LCC HQ767.9 .J33 2023 (print) | LCC HQ767.9 (ebook) | DDC
    305.231–dc23/eng/20230417
LC record available at https://lccn.loc.gov/2023009374
LC ebook record available at https://lccn.loc.gov/2023009375

ISBN 979-8-88770-061-8 paperback
ISBN 979-8-88770-062-5 ePub

Printed in the United States of America

First edition: 2023

For Morgan and Drew.
As a parent my wish for you is a life lived
to the fullest and surrounded by love.

To Doug, my parents, sisters, in-laws,
and friends who have become family.
The Harvard Happiness Study taught us
that our connections and community bring
us fulfillment. My life is filled with joy, laughter,
and love through these relationships.
I love you all.

To the Brain Balance community of kids,
parents, adults, and colleagues. You have taught
me more than any classroom ever could.

CONTENTS

HOW TO READ THIS BOOK

Grab a highlighter and a pen as you begin to read this book. I recommend resisting the urge to jump ahead to the passages that apply most to your current concerns. Development is a complex process, and a child who is on track in many areas can still be behind in others. Don't assume that because your child is older, they have achieved all the milestones set out in the sections targeted at younger kids. Start at the beginning and work your way forward. What you'll learn throughout this book is that critical aspects of early foundational development contribute to your overarching goals for your child. By reading through the book in its entirety, you will walk away with a deeper understanding of your child's development and how to support the area of concern that prompted you to buy this book in the first place. Reading past your child's current age will help you know what to anticipate in the coming years and may also spark both a deeper understanding and additional brainstorms for helping your child and family along the way.

As you read through the developmental milestones in each section, check off the milestones your child has achieved. Then, with your highlighter, note the next milestones to work toward achieving.

In the activities section in each chapter, highlight activities you haven't done and that would be a good fit for your child.

Next, create your action plan. Reviewing the categories in which you highlighted gaps in development, and activities to support these gaps, will help you map a plan for progress. It isn't realistic to do everything every day, so creating a plan for each month will allow you to hit on many key areas on different days and weeks.

Finally, track your child's progress over time. When you revisit the milestones sections after several months have passed, use a different color pen to begin to check off new milestones your child is achieving. Development is not perfectly linear but happens in bursts and plateaus, and each new stage of development can also include new challenges as kids test boundaries and explore their expanding abilities. This can be stressful and doesn't always feel like forward momentum. Tracking the newly achieved milestones can be an important visual reminder that progress is being made.

Powerful change and progress can and will happen with a consistent approach for support and integrating activities into your daily lifestyle; however, this book is not meant as a replacement for other services. The **activities, guidance, and suggestions in this book can be integrated before and after completing the Brain Balance program or other services or approaches that support developmental gains and success.**

BACK ON TRACK

INTRODUCTION

• • • •

THE PANDEMIC AND DEVELOPMENT

As parents, one of our greatest stressors in life is ensuring the well-being of our kids.

Is my daughter okay? Is she happy? Will she make good choices in life that keep her away from harm and trouble? Is she getting along with friends? Does she feel a sense of belonging and confidence in who she is?

Will my son be strong enough to stand up to peer pressure, to do what is right in life, even when it is hard? Is he keeping up in school, getting his work turned in? Will he live in my basement for the rest of his life?

Are their struggles behavioral, or is there something more going on with my child? Are they acting out on purpose for attention? Am I not parenting this child in the way they need? Do I need to change my discipline approach, the school they are in, or how I motivate and encourage them? What am I doing wrong, and why is this so hard?

Every generation faces versions of these questions and concerns. But not every generation has faced the additional challenges today's kids and parents are facing after over a year of remote school, two years of wearing masks in public, and massive levels of stress, fear, and change that disrupted a significant portion of growing years. The events of the pandemic and the ongoing ripple effects are what sparked my motivation to write *Back on Track*, but the information in this book applies to the development of all kids, with or without a pandemic. These last few years simply acted as a catalyst and reminder of what we know about the key drivers and supports for development.

This book is for every parent who has worried about their child and wants to know how they can help their child thrive. The chapters in this book will help you better understand why stress, change, and disruption in daily experiences impact our kids' *development* and how they *feel* and *function*. This deeper understanding will allow you to connect the dots between what *is* and what *could be* and *why*. Even more importantly, this book will provide insights and tools you can begin to implement today, for kids of all ages.

This book is not about understanding the array of diagnoses and labels that can apply to kids, but about understanding the many developmental nuances that contribute to children's growth and development. For example, struggles with attention are a part of ADHD and can also be experienced with anxiety, autism, and a sensory processing disorder. Immaturity in physical coordination is a hallmark of a developmental coordination disorder, as well as of autism and ADHD. Disruptions in sensory processing can impact anxiety and the development of emotional maturity.

The symptoms and challenges parents encounter daily are not specific to one diagnosis but impact an array of aspects in life. By focusing on the underlying functions that support healthy development, you can focus on the child in front of you rather than on the label. I'm not suggesting that a diagnosis is not important, or necessary, but that the foundational developmental areas discussed in this book are larger than any one label, impacting all kids and their growth in many areas.

The far-reaching impact of an understanding of the fundamentals of development has been one of the most important takeaways I've experienced in my career, and other people's lack of awareness—even other professionals working with kids—has been a frustration. As parents, teachers, and healthcare professionals, it's easy to focus on the biggest symptom—whatever is causing the most pain, discomfort, or disruption to life—and miss the underlying causation and the broader impact. The child who melts down daily and disrupts the classroom, dinnertime, or bedtime is often seen as a behavioral challenge. But the reality may be a hypersensitivity to sensory stimuli, a lack of coordination, or immaturity in impulse control. Understanding the overlap and interplay of the many aspects of development, and how that contributes to the goal—better behavior, for example—can provide a more efficient path to success.

Imagine you're a parent of a struggling ten-year-old boy, and you are trying to understand what is going on with your child and how to help. You may wait six months for an appointment for an evaluation and possible diagnosis, and then at the end of the day the child may or may not meet the threshold for ADHD. There can be relief in that moment: "phew, he doesn't have ADHD." Or, alternatively, "he does have ADHD, which can provide an explanation for the challenges I've been facing." But now, there is also confusion and ambiguity. If he does have ADHD, you need to consider options to help: medication, behavior management, or an approach to create change in the brain. If he doesn't have ADHD, you will be left with questions of what *is* going on and what you can do to help.

The reality is that the difference between a child being diagnosed with ADHD or not may come down to the parent's answer on one question in a list of questions designed to help diagnose ADHD. If the child falls one question short of reaching the threshold, do they still struggle? Yes. Are that parent's concerns still real and valid? Absolutely. Is that child still experiencing complications that are disrupting learning, peer and family relationships, and their behavior? Yup. This child may be struggling a little less than other kids who do meet the threshold for the diagnosis, but the challenge is still present, and a plan of action and support is still needed.

It's easy to look at a label or diagnosis as very black and white, and in some instances it is. A cancer diagnosis, for example, is usually more straightforward: you have it or you don't. But with developmental concerns and disorders, there are many shades of gray along an entire spectrum of development.

In this book, the question isn't "Do they have *it*?" (ADHD, a sensory processing disorder, a learning disability, autism, anxiety, etc.). The question is, "Are things harder than they need to be?" And, if the answer to that is yes, next ask yourself, "If there was improvement around the concern, would there be a benefit to my child? To our family and home environment?" If you answered yes to any of these questions, this book is for you.

One frequent question I get from parents is, "Will they outgrow it?" The very direct answer is, "most likely, no." The challenge will evolve and change over time, but the underlying complication creating the behavior, the struggle with socializing or learning, often persists. The eight-year-old falling out of their seat in class won't be a thirty-eight-year-old falling out of their chair at work but probably will be struggling more with time management, with controlling their temper when stressed or frustrated, and with execution of more complex tasks, even if they have high intelligence. The child who hates socks and tags in clothing will keep their socks and shoes on as an adult but may be more irritable after a day in a loud and chaotic environment and may struggle more with sustained attention and anxiety.

This doesn't mean they can't or won't be successful; it means in some areas they will need to work harder and use more compensatory strategies to help them succeed. ADHD, for example, was previously described as a childhood disorder and is now classified as a life span disorder. It usually doesn't go away, but as adults we get better at compensating for our challenges. My advice is: Don't wait to see if next year looks different from this year. Let's work to drive change rather than make a lifetime of compensation. If you have a concern, act now.

Chances are, if you're paging through this book, you're at a point of stress and frustration. Something needs to change, but it's hard to know what to do and where to begin. Maybe this is your first stop, and you're just starting to dig deeper to try and understand what is going on with your child, or maybe you've been searching and working for years to support your child's growth and well-being. Even if you've already done an entire list of programs and services, change is still possible. If the ideas and suggestions in this book are different from what you've done in the past, then there is the potential for the outcomes to be different as well. If sections in this book resonate with what you've been experiencing, know that change is possible. The brain is incredibly complex and constantly evolving. An increased understanding of what drives development and a specialized plan to purposefully exercise and engage the brain can make a difference. Children are amazingly resilient, and with the right knowledge and support, getting them back on track can be as simple as adding some specific and intentional activities to your daily routine to advance brain pathways for development.

Change is a process that won't happen overnight, but the purposeful work and education you commit to now has the potential to positively impact your child every day going forward.

Pandemic Lessons

Even prior to March 2020, far too many kids and adults were struggling with regulating focus, mood, anxiety, stress levels, organization, comprehension, and more. Then the pandemic hit, and it became an amplifier of all challenges. You struggled with focus? It became a bigger uphill battle. Anxiety? It got worse. Keeping up in class or at work was hard? It just got even harder. Organizing your time and making important decisions? They became even more draining to accomplish.

I saw instantly how the shifts we made impacted the daily lives and demeanors of my own kids, Morgan and Drew. Their natural initial reaction of fear and uncertainty morphed into boredom, loneliness, and sluggishness. Their days of social interaction, school, and sports came to a screeching halt. They began spending more time than ever on the couch or in their bedrooms with the doors closed. More time on their devices. Less time with friends and less time being physically active. New and different demands began cropping up: log into a Zoom meeting for the first time, learn how to navigate school through a computer, download pdfs, submit schoolwork online. Attempt to manage your time while parents juggle their own demands at work from the kitchen table or room next door. *As fourth and sixth graders.*

The demands and challenges were obvious, and they were an understandable reaction to the new and evolving crisis the world was facing, but that didn't lessen the impact.

As more time passed and the data and research began to emerge, it became increasingly evident that the pandemic and its fallout would have more than a minor impact on our children. And while life has moved on from remote learning and social distancing, we are still discovering the impact the changes that took place during this time had on our kids. Increased rates of anxiety, depression, and ADHD. A widening academic achievement gap. Higher rates of disruption and violence in the classroom.

Every child from birth on up was affected to some degree by our sustained pandemic response, regardless of whether there was a pre-existing concern. It wasn't just our kids with ADHD or anxiety or our teenagers suffering the consequences; all kids were impacted to varying degrees.

It is critical to note that the impact goes deeper than simply a change to our moods and emotions. Science is showing that actual structural changes occurred in the brains of infants born during this time. Infants as young as six months old are testing behind in gross motor skills, fine motor skills, and communication.[1] The four- to seven-year-olds at Brain Balance, a comprehensive program designed to engage and strengthen the brain to minimize challenges, experienced a 15% drop in fine motor skills, and children ages four to seventeen were struggling more with tasks involving timing with auditory and visual processing. Parents are reporting greater concerns with their kids' mood and emotions, as well as concerns with their reading, writing, and math abilities. School-age children fell behind academically, with even more alarming rates of decline in low-income socioeconomic regions,[2] and teens have been experiencing unprecedented rates of anxiety, depression, and suicide.[3] Nearly three years after the start of the pandemic, the Nation's Report Card, the largest national ongoing measure of K–12 education and how much kids are learning, indicates staggering levels of decline in reading and math scores, backsliding on decades of progress.[4]

Parents are grappling with concerns and with finding the path forward to support their kids: "Is my child struggling in school now because of two years of distance learning, or is there something more going on? What can or should I be doing to help?"

There is not a country that I'm aware of that has not experienced ramifications of COVID, beyond the direct health impact. This leaves us with approximately 72 million babies born into the pandemic in 2020, and *hundreds of millions of children* around the world, who experienced several years of their critical developmental years during the pandemic crisis response.

While the world has moved beyond the time of social distancing and remote school, we need to learn from the past to support our future. Beyond the need to learn how to address the pandemic development dip, the fallout from this time has become a resounding reminder of what our kids need to thrive in their growth and development.

The mission of this book is to create an understanding and offer an action plan for all parents to get kids back on track for the brightest future possible. No one escaped the pandemic unscathed, and everyone will experience future times of stress and disruption in life. **Knowing how stress, change, and daily experiences affect our ability to regulate focus, mood, and behavior will help parents develop a path forward to make a positive difference in their children's development and lives.**

Like millions around the world, my family had to shift how our home and family functioned beginning in March 2020. We hunkered down to weather the rapidly unfolding crisis; we were all spending more time than ever on devices and less time moving and interacting. Understanding the brain, I *knew* this was problematic for the well-being of all of us, but most of all for my kids (ages ten and twelve at the time the pandemic began).

Reducing physical activity, experiences, and engagement lessens the refinement and development of brain connectivity—impacting perception, language, cognition, and social/emotional development.

The more immature the brain is developmentally, the *less* it is able to pay attention, control mood and emotion, learn, interact, and execute. These functions evolve as a result of brain development. Adrienne Tierney of the Harvard Graduate School of Education in the scientific journal *Zero Three* describes brain development as the formation and refinement of neural networks.[5] The refinement of these brain pathways involves building new connections, pruning nonessential ones, and improving speed, complexity, and precision. These network changes in the brain are essential to maturation and happen over time through use and challenge. "The foundations of sensory and perceptual systems that are critical to language, social behavior, and emotion are formed in the early years and are strongly influenced by experiences during this time."[6] **Development is the result of improved brain connectivity.**

This means that the new hurdles we were all facing because of the pandemic were impeding the use of and challenge to brain pathways as a result of reduced exposure to a variety of new and different stimuli and experiences. Kids need to continue to refine their neural networks to mature their skills and abilities—to drive the process of developing the brain. This time of prolonged stress and change was challenging for adults, but it was having an even bigger impact on our kids.

This concern was constantly in the background of my thoughts. And I was driving my kids nuts. Put down the phone. Go outside. Go for a run, walk, bike ride. *Anything.* Move, do *something* outside this house to protect your brain, your development, and your well-being.

In the meantime, at Brain Balance, a company whose programs are designed to engage the brain to enhance cognition, development, and emotional well-being, we were receiving more calls than ever from parents worried about their child's anxiety, lack of attention, meltdowns, and moods. Doing school from home increased many parents' awareness of some of the struggles their kids were already experiencing—add to that the pandemic complications, and nearly every struggle intensified. Each month that passed we were seeing an escalation in these concerns. And while the crisis response was shifting over time, the calls from parents weren't slowing down.

All this was churning in my awareness, but it was one unexpected interaction that brought the significance of this time in our lives to a head for me.

I spent one morning with a local photographer, Susan, shooting photos. My professional headshots were outdated and in desperate need of a revamp. I love this particular photographer because of her knack for putting you at ease during an awkward experience, capturing real expressions and moments. She does this by keeping up a constant stream of chatter and finding topics you are passionate about discussing. This of course led to a conversation around the pandemic and the impact on our kids.

Susan shared that as early as December 2020, she had started to notice a change in the babies she was photographing for their one-year-old pictures. Even though she had been doing this successfully for years, shoot after shoot did not go well. Pictures weren't turning out and needed to be redone. Babies were fussy, uncooperative, and wanting to be held by Mom.

She ultimately put a new policy in place. Prior to scheduling your baby's photo session, you needed to spend time with your baby outside your home. The babies needed to see people other than immediate family so they weren't scared of her or the camera. Parents needed to be able to set their child on the floor with a toy and walk away. All things that sounded simple and inconsequential, but all things that demonstrated to me just how much life had changed for these 2020 babies in a matter of mere months.

Susan nailed it: The babies were different in their development and interactions. She saw the immediate impact of the past year, but what did it mean for these kids going forward?

While my concern had been for my own kids and family, I had neglected to truly consider the ramification for babies and what this meant for the disruption of their foundational development.

We were facing not only a pandemic crisis but a developmental crisis in our youth.

I raced home to begin scouring the internet for research. What *did* we know about the impact that was occurring? What had we learned from previous periods of prolonged stress for pregnant mothers about the subsequent development of their infants? What had we already measured that could help us understand current development impacts, well-being impacts, and academic skills impacts?

While there was already some knowledge and data, the conversation was focused on discussing and defining the concerns. But where was the conversation on what to do to help? Where was the critical messaging and guidance to support parents and help our kids?

This critical conversation can't happen quickly or loudly enough. We need as many experts and authorities as possible weighing in on this matter, contributing to help an entire generation of kids thrive as we move beyond this tumultuous time.

While I certainly do not have all the answers, my education and experiences have equipped me with the means to not only define and understand the challenges but also to provide parents with the tools to help support the development and well-being of their kids.

Science over the past few decades has taught us that the brain can change. It's never too late to strengthen the networks in the brain that support how you feel and function. Creating a plan to stimulate and engage your child's brain and body will help forge a better way forward.

No parent wants to watch their child struggle or hurt, and we'll go to great lengths to help. Yet, the most convenient approach is not always the most beneficial. We live in a culture that often focuses on symptoms, not causes. If you have a headache, pop an Advil. The headache may go away, but do you understand what caused the headache in the first place? Maybe you were dehydrated, hungry, or tired. If you knew what was contributing to the headache, you could focus on the underlying issue that resulted in the symptom.

Our kids will benefit from us applying this same philosophy to their challenges. If the struggle is attention, instead of approaching it like a behavior, we need to look to the underlying brain connections that control attention. Digging deeper to understand why attention is lacking gives us an opportunity to positively impact a child's attentional development by building and refining the pathways that support attention.

Everything we do is orchestrated by the brain, an enormously complex and intricate organ we are only beginning to understand. Development involves changes in the brain's pathways—new experiences form new connections in the brain, helping us learn and grow in our abilities. Each skill we have requires its own neural network; to do something complex requires *many* separate networks all firing in perfect harmony to create the desired outcome. While it's easy to observe the outcome—the ability to read, pay attention, or control your mood and behavior—it isn't easy to observe the individual network that coordinates with other networks to contribute to the whole.

A disruption in experiences that lead to the building of these pathways makes it harder for our kids to do the things expected of them. A study published in *Molecular Psychiatry* in 2022 illustrates how certain brain tasks are more difficult for kids with ADHD, a disorder that involves immaturity in brain connectivity. The study found that kids with ADHD struggled more with neural flexibility—the ability to multi-task or switch from task to task.[7] The result is a child who is working on homework and becomes distracted by an alert on their phone, so they grab their phone to check it—and forget to return to the original task. Brain imaging in this study showed specifically that pathways in the brain involved with sensory, motor, and visual functions were impacted in kids with ADHD.

More simply put—disorganization in the brain's networks results in disorganization in outcomes, and disorganization in outcomes can be an indicator of disorganization in the brain. These outcomes can impact mood, behavior, attention, learning, and social interactions. Kids who experience fluctuations in their behaviors and abilities from day to day, who struggle to complete a task without prompting or have a smaller threshold for frustrations and upsets, are all showing signs of possible immaturity, or disorganization, in brain pathways. The result is that these kids must work harder than their peers to accomplish a task. On the days they are well rested and well fed and have fewer distractions, parents can see a glimmer of what their children are truly capable of accomplishing. The challenge is that a child may not be able to repeat good behavior or a desired performance day after day, and may find themselves drained and irritable more frequently. It all starts in the brain. To have organized thoughts and actions, you need organized brain connections.

This may sound daunting, but change is possible. Brain development is a lifelong process. Refinement continues to happen in our neural pathways from use and challenge.[8] Going back to the basics to ensure a stronger foundation of networks and pathways can help contribute to a better organization of pathways in the brain, culminating in improved skills, functions, and consistency of abilities.

Lakshmi was a perfect example of a child who appeared to be experiencing disorganization in key developmental pathways. This disruption created a problematic symptom—struggles with reading. And while the family was focused on the symptom, the underlying complication, the disorganized brain pathways that support reading, had never been addressed.

Lakshmi was in kindergarten when the pandemic hit. The first part of the year went well, and she enjoyed school. Then the year ended early, and Lakshmi had over five months off from school. Her entire first-grade year was remote. In addition to the challenge of virtual school for a six-year-old, the teacher changed mid-year. Her parents tried to help with worksheets and activities but were also juggling working from home. When second grade resumed in person with masks, it was a huge relief to everyone, but that relief didn't last long. Lakshmi started complaining about school and not wanting to go. The work was hard for her, and she knew it. Her parents were flooded with guilt. She'd had so much disruption between the pandemic and change in teachers, and they felt like they'd let things fall between the cracks for their daughter's learning.

Testing early in the year flagged Lakshmi's reading at nearly two years behind. Her mom shared that she was shocked at how far behind Lakshmi was testing. "I felt like such a failure. I knew she didn't like reading, but I had no idea how much she was struggling. Immediately we started practicing more each night, and that was a nightmare. School started the process of assessing her to identify needs for support services, but the process was slow. We did an online phonics program. She made some improvements, but I worried she was continuing to fall even further behind."

The family reached out to Brain Balance for help, and I quickly noted that in talking with Lakshmi, it was evident that she was bright. In fact, when we tested her auditory comprehension, she scored 90% on a second-grade passage—right on track for her age and grade. When we switched gears to reading comprehension questions after trying to read a simple passage, the result was dismal—but it provided key information. She did great until she needed to use her eyes. But this wasn't about needing glasses to see clearly. Her assessment showed that Lakshmi's eyes were all over the place as she read—jumping, skipping, bouncing all around. Brain Balance utilizes eye-tracking technology to better understand eye movements, coordination, and processing, and a live simulation allows you to see the precise eye movements while tracking a dot or reading a passage. Lakshmi's eyes would overshoot or under-shoot the target and would move in an inconsistent pattern, resulting in extra movements that were inefficient. I could see it as well in simply having Lakshmi track my finger slowly from side to side. Her eyes didn't move smoothly to track.

Lakshmi didn't have a comprehension challenge; she struggled with eye movements, accuracy, and processing. Her eyes jumped and skipped, moving *more* in a short passage than the eyes of other kids her age. She was working harder, with lower outcomes. She perceived words and word parts out of order and missed some words altogether. Her comprehension was low and her reading laborious because of disorganized eye movements. Her *symptom* was delayed reading, but the *underlying mechanism* appeared to be the lack of maturity in the pathways that control the coordination of eye movements. These movements are supported by networks in the brain that control precision, efficiency, endurance, and processing and typically improve over time through development.

After working a chain of developmental events with Lakshmi—that included key categories we will discuss throughout this book—she experienced huge gains quickly. She ended the school year on track with her reading.

The best part about Lakshmi's gains was how they impacted her image of herself. She went from feeling stupid to feeling capable. Her parents saw a big shift in her confidence.

Learning was impacted for Lakshmi because of a disruption in her foundational development, and when that development was strengthened, the work she put into learning was more efficient and effective.

While Lakshmi experienced an obvious disruption in her exposure and development, that's not the case for all kids. Some kids demonstrate symptoms and challenges without an obvious reason for a disruption in their development. The good news is that regardless of *why* a child presents immaturity and disorganization in skills and behaviors, the brain can benefit from specific exercises and activities designed to support refining brain networks and drive healthy development.

The brain is complex beyond our ability to comprehend. There is no need to feel guilty or bad as a parent if your child has challenges. The reality is that all brains have strengths *and* areas that would benefit from targeted exercises to improve performance. It's also true that disruptions in development *amplify* existing concerns and can result in additional challenges. But those challenges will bring attention to areas that you have the opportunity to help. So rather than stressing about the concerns, use that information to guide you, like a flashlight shining ahead to show you the best path forward.

What has become very clear to me over the course of my career is that while parents have a great understanding of what development looks like from in utero until age two, there isn't a good understanding of what development looks like in an older child. It's also easy to miss how interconnected challenges may be. **Nothing in the brain happens in isolation—an immaturity in one area will impact other areas.** In fact, one neuron in the brain can connect to up to 1,000 other neurons. The student who struggles with attention may also struggle to manage their behaviors and to eat a variety of foods without a battle or meltdown. The child who battles anxiety may also be clumsy and dislike tags on clothing. While these may *feel* like separate issues to a parent, these pathways all directly or indirectly contribute to executive functions. The bottom line is that a child's cognitive and executive function abilities—attention, memory, learning, organization, and goal management—are tied to brain development. The more we know about these core functions, the better we can support these areas.

In 2018, after being a Brain Balance center owner with my husband for a decade, I was asked to join the executive team to help evolve and expand the program offerings—to update and adapt our program based on current research findings. With a focus on research, results, and outcomes, I now had the opportunity to see and learn from the data on a much broader scale. At Brain Balance we have assessed over 150,000 people. Digging into this extensive data helped me to understand how *functional* abilities such as balance, coordination, timing, and eye movements are the result of brain networks. Looking to these functional skills can provide insights into brain connectivity and maturity. Leveraging this understanding of how brain connections and abilities are connected also provides a path for using specialized exercises and activities to refine the neural pathways to optimize development. As parents we have the opportunity to engage and exercise our kids' brains to influence their development. As I shifted from a center owner to an executive team member at Brain Balance, I also shifted gears in my ongoing professional coursework, next digging further into research.

From the George Washington University Medical School program on clinical translational research, I learned that only a fraction of published research (an estimated 14%) ever makes it into the mainstream programs and protocols utilized by schools, physicians, and others, and when it does, it can take an average of *seventeen years* before these findings are applied.[9] The parent in me was sick at heart to hear this statistic. A struggling child can't wait seventeen years for an intervention that could potentially help them succeed. My focus became *translational research,* which aims to shorten the process from learning to implementation—to move research findings more quickly into practice. Through this approach with Brain Balance, I've published research on changes in cognition, attention, behavior, and emotions to improve a child's ability to learn, grow, and interact positively with the world around them.

When the pandemic hit, I watched changes in the data. Kids were presenting with larger gaps in some areas than they had been pre-pandemic. To me this reinforced the importance of the fundamentals of childhood: sensory exposure, play, physical activity, group and social learning, and experiences. Hopefully this generation will not need to experience another pandemic, but we can apply what we've learned to meet the immediate needs of our youth and to better support kids going forward.

I've traveled extensively to seek out the latest advances in technology, research, and cognition. To see what is being developed in research labs to both measure and impact the brain—for kids, the aging population, and even professional athletes. From tech coming out of Stanford to gamified cognitive tools from the University of California at San Francisco to industry technology being developed for kids, athletes, and aging adults both in the United States and internationally, the common denominator is the brain and what can be done to exercise and engage pathways in a way to improve performance—whether at home, in the classroom, in the boardroom, with friends, or on the playing field.

I have sought to meet and learn from as many *different* experts as I could in a variety of fields that all directly impact the brain: psychology, neurology, cognition, pediatrics, physical therapy, occupational therapy, education, kinesiology, functional neurology, nutrition, and more. My goal has been to surround myself with people far smarter than me, to continue learning and growing.

I feel the answer to helping kids (and adults) thrive doesn't rely on any *one* of these fields but on *all* these fields. It has been through these collaborations and experiences that I've had the privilege of working to create programs for kids, adults, and athletes—in centers and from home—all with outcomes of improved well-being, cognition, and performance.

Back on Track is a culmination of two decades of learning, practice, and research paired with observations from pandemic times that highlighted to me what is needed to maximize development and well-being. My sincere wish is to share with you information and strategies that I've learned through experience and research that have impacted my life in the hopes it has an impact on those you love as well.

1

• • • •

COORDINATION DEVELOPMENT

As parents, we're stuck in a continual conundrum. We try not to compare our children to their siblings or other kids. Yet those observations and comparisons are some of the main ways we set benchmarks to determine if our kids are on track, ahead, or behind.

While each child is unique—and this should be celebrated—there are numerous milestones that are expected to be achieved by certain ages for development to be considered on track. These markers have been set by the Centers for Disease Control and other professional groups and indicate what the majority of kids are able to achieve at each age. These milestones are guideposts that let us know when our children are developing as expected and when they're lagging behind.

Neural pathways in the brain refine over time to become faster and more complex—this refinement creates pathways that fire with greater ease, efficiency, and complexity, which matures the functions they support. That's why this chapter is all about starting with the basics to build a foundation for your child to excel. This foundation is critical as later development depends on early development.[1]

Picture a marionette—a puppet that can only dance when its strings are pulled. The brain is like the puppeteer, pulling the strings and controlling the coordination of our movements, perceptions, and actions.

Movement and coordination milestones can be some of the easiest to observe, but it's also easy to underestimate their importance. If physical coordination is on track, that is a good indicator that the neural pathways that control muscles and coordination are on track. For example, if an eighteen-month-old is able to walk without holding on to anyone or anything and can climb on and off a couch or chair without help, this is an indicator of age-appropriate development of physical coordination. If coordination is not on track, this is an indicator that other regions in the brain and related development will be impacted.

The complexity of development and the intricate interplay between neurons and their functions are why at Brain Balance we created our own parent survey tool. We needed to understand more about each child. The standard tools focus on one area of concern at a time. This approach provides important input about that area but not about the full child and the scope of impact on multiple areas. If a child has concerns or delays in one developmental area, the odds are extremely high there will be an impact in other areas of development as well. To understand more about the whole child, we were asking parents hundreds of questions using multiple tools, which wasn't efficient. Using the existing database of questions and data allowed us to create a new survey tool covering multiple domains of development in one survey. The Brain Balance Multi-Domain Developmental Survey (which is available to view in the published study) works to get a sense of developmental strengths and areas for concern in one scientifically validated tool.[2] To fully understand a child's development, the focus needs to be not just on the main area of parent concern but on the whole child: their attention, academics, behavior, anxiety, social interactions, coordination, sensory processing, impulsivity, and more.

For kids who are neurodivergent, whose development is delayed due to genetics, pathology, or other reasons, parents can struggle to know how their children are developing relative to others with a similar condition. For example, age-based milestones don't exist specific to disorders or conditions. This impacts a wide array of conditions, including Down syndrome, Fragile X, Klinefelter syndrome, and others, including autism. This can leave parents in the dark about how their children are progressing relative to other kids with the same condition, or what next steps to take to support them. While the timeline for achieving milestones may look different for some neurodivergent children, you can still find a starting point that is appropriate for your child and use the exercises and activities in this book to purposefully engage their brain. Growth and forward momentum are meaningful at every age and ability. Know that completing the activities in this book won't enable all kids to overcome all challenges, but there is value in a purposeful action plan to support your child's unique levels of development. Just as everyone benefits from nutrition and exercise, we all benefit from stimulation and movement designed to strengthen connections in the brain. As you use this book, focus less on your child's current age and more on the milestones they have or haven't yet achieved to guide your unique starting point and journey.

All development starts simply and builds in complexity. Kids start with simple gestures, such as waving bye-bye. But through a chain of events that occur over time, movements become highly complex, nuanced patterns of action and interaction with the world—beginning with rolling and crawling, evolving into the ability to drive a car, to dance the rumba (who does that anymore?), to make a fancy dinner, to type a book manuscript, or to build a new deck. These activities all depend on coordinated movements and timing to be successful. And while many parents aren't worried about their child's core muscle strength and basic coordination, it's often because they underestimate the importance of these elements. Higher-level functions are dependent on lower-level functions.[3]

Bottom line—don't skip this crucial chapter! You'll learn something to help you more fully understand the symptoms and concerns that prompted you to pick up this book in the first place. In fact, cognitive development is dependent on motor development. One example of this is a study that found **that a delay in early motor and language milestones between 3 and 18 months was correlated with a higher incidence of learning challenges and ADHD.**[4] Movement and coordination matter for all kids.

Note to Parents

To help you find opportunities to springboard your child's development ahead, I'm giving you permission to observe and compare your child's movements and coordination at all ages—not just the toddler years—without guilt. If the other kids in the neighborhood are riding bikes and your child isn't, note this. If your child is fifteen months old and not yet walking, you can help. In gymnastics class when the kids do jumping jacks and your child is out of sync, this is useful information for you. Avoiding sports and physical activities isn't the answer. You can help your child fill in those gaps.

If you don't have other kids as comparisons for your child's abilities, simply use the milestone sections in this book to determine areas of focus to drive the next development steps.

Remember that coordination is not only about learning to crawl and walk. It's an important factor at every age and every stage. All too often I hear parents make excuses for their kids like "He's just not sporty" or "She's more of a book kid." That may be true, and books are awesome, but remember that even reading, writing, and engineering require several brain networks coordinating to perform intricate movements and timing—all of which begin with the basic fundamentals developed in childhood.

No more excuses, no more guilt. The pandemic taught us that coordination and development are impacted when activities and interactions change. During lockdowns, kids had fewer opportunities for play, sports, and movement, and we *know* that for far too many kids, this impacted their development of coordination. We can't fight that reality, but we can put an action plan in place to help ensure healthy development for our kids moving forward.

Pandemic Lessons

The science journal *Nature* published pandemic-related research in January 2022 that focused on infant development. The study found that at just six months of age, babies born during the pandemic were already *behind* in key areas of development: gross motor skills, fine motor skills, and communication.[5] This was staggering news. These babies were already affected by the changes in how we were living day to day that had an impact on their muscles, coordination, and movement. "We're in a crisis, I don't know what to do, because we not only have an effect of a pandemic, but it's a significant one," shared Morgan Firestein, a postdoctoral researcher at Columbia University.[6]

Other labs studying infant development observed the same thing. "[Assessment s]cores during the pandemic were much worse than those from previous years. Things just began sort of falling off a rock at the tail end of last year and the beginning part of this year," said Sean Deoni, a medical biophysicist at Brown University's Advanced Baby Imaging Lab in Providence, Rhode Island, in late 2021. The research clearly indicated that babies born during the first year of the pandemic scored slightly lower than pre-pandemic infants on developmental screening tests. Deoni also noted "the longer the pandemic has continued, the more deficits children have accumulated. The magnitude is massive—it's just astonishing."[7]

You may be asking yourself, what can a baby even *do* at six months regarding these areas of development? The Ages and Stages Questionnaires, or the ASQ–3, the screening tools used in the study cited in *Nature,* evaluated if a baby at six months had the gross motor ability to do tasks such as straightening both arms to push their chest off the floor when lying on their tummy, rolling from back to tummy, sitting while leaning forward and resting their weight on their arms, and lifting their legs high enough to see their feet when lying on their back.

These movements may seem simple, almost inconsequential, but they're anything but minor in the grand scheme of development. Many studies have correlated early motor performance (birth to four years old) with later cognitive performance (ages six to eleven years). Motor performance is a predictor for academic and cognitive abilities, including attention.[8] Those early motor milestones matter.

For infants, engaging core muscles through tummy time is critical. For toddlers, running, playing, and exploring are foundational to their growth in coordination. For older kids, the brain needs daily physical activities to drive learning and growth. Even as adults, the brain craves movement to enhance our levels of focus and mood. Yet statistics that tracked activities of families during the pandemic showed less time spent engaging core muscles, running, moving, or playing and more time—you guessed it—engaged with technology.

Using more technology didn't only affect teens and adults. There was a direct impact in babies younger than one year, because rather than having lots of face-to-face interactions with infants in the family, parents and siblings were glued to their devices. The *New York Times* reported that internet use among kids had doubled since pre-pandemic use as early as May 2020, and it continued to increase over time. "What concerns researchers, at a minimum, is that the use of devices is a poor substitute for activities known to be central to health, social and physical development, including physical play and other interactions that help children learn how to confront challenging social situations."[9] Not only does this lack of movement impact development, but increased digital usage impacts other aspects of overall health and well-being, including mood, energy, and even sleep.[10]

But don't feel guilty about the past! We all did what we needed to do to get through a stressful and surreal time. But now, armed with facts and a plan, you can fire up your child's brain, development, and overall well-being, and you can do this whether they're ahead, on track, or behind.

All development begins simply and evolves to become more complex with experience and repetition as the brain and body learn control and timing. Then, as development continues, you learn to integrate complex movement with other skills, such as sensory information, thought, and even the planning and execution of highly complex tasks. To become coordinated, your brain must synchronize several separate regions of the brain and body with precise timing.

Picture a hockey player and consider all the elements of coordination involved in a single play. To try to score a goal, the player may need to skate around another player and pass the puck to an open teammate to set them up to score. Skating and stick handling require coordination, and there's tons of sensory input as the player watches what's happening around him and thinks about and plans his next move. And this entire sequence of coordinated events happens in only a second or two.

But we don't start life with this intricate design of all the elements of coordination. We begin with one coordinated task at a time. Then as we improve, our coordination evolves to become more complex and precise, simultaneously involving more and more separate components. And it all begins by first developing our core muscles and learning simple coordination.

Science Alert

Within the brain, there's a bundle of nerves whose functions directly dictate our levels of alertness, muscle tone, and the varying amounts of sensory information the brain takes in at any given moment. This is the reticular acti-vating system, or RAS for short.

If you've ever wondered why you feel so tired after a day of just sitting around, or why when there's a crash in the night, you're instantly awake and on high alert, it's because of the RAS.

The job of the RAS is to regulate many things, including behavior, arousal (level of wakefulness versus sleep), consciousness, and your ability to focus.[11] Your awareness then guides your behaviors and responses to the information the brain receives. The primary job of this system is to act as the gate between your senses and your brain, controlling how much information you are receiv-ing at any given time. When you're asleep, this system closes the gate. This decreases the amount of sensory information you process, which helps you to fall asleep and stay that way. The sensory info is still there: the temperature in the room, the dog barking outside, the darkness, the weight of your blankets. Your brain is simply not processing that information while you sleep. And when it's time to wake up, the RAS reopens the gate to increase your levels of alert-ness and to allow you to take in more sensory information so you can orient yourself and interact with the world.

The RAS can be activated in many different ways. Think about the alarm clock that jars you from a restful sleep. You roll over and silence the alarm as quickly as possible. Next, as you slowly begin to wake up, you stretch. This movement stretches your spinal cord and the muscles that support your spine and posture, activating the RAS, which sends signals to fire up and wake your brain. The spinal cord and supporting muscles signal to the brain to wake up and pay attention, and to start taking in sensory information.

If your alarm clock is really loud, or if there's some other loud stimulus, you awaken with a jolt. That jolt is the RAS turning on with a bang from being activated through the fight or flight startle response. Your brain is now instan-taneously on high alert. You're taking in as much information as possible and trying to determine what woke you, if there's danger, or if any action is needed. Your muscle tone is high, and your brain and body are ready for anything. A high-stress response prodded the RAS to go into high drive and to hyper focus on potentially relevant information.[12]

Do you remember your teachers telling you, "Sit up to pay attention!"? Are you starting to connect the dots about why sitting up straight helps you to focus? You guessed it; it's the RAS. Stretching your spinal cord and engaging the postural core muscles increases activation. It signals your brain to increase attention and increase awareness of your senses.

Infants and Toddlers

We've talked about achieving developmental milestones, so let's take a look at various recommendations. While I was writing this book, an unusual event took place that changed how parents and professionals talk about developmental milestones. The Centers for Disease Control (CDC), which defines developmental milestones, revised its decades-old guidelines. This was very unexpected and created a cascade of thoughts and opinions on the changes from parents and professionals alike. The CDC's stated goal is to help parents more clearly identify when a child is behind in each area. Previous recommendations stated the ages at which 50% of kids were accomplishing the milestone. Updated guidelines have shifted to 75% of kids. This means that most kids can achieve that milestone by the listed age, and if your child has not, they are falling in the lower 25% of kids on that task, a red flag for concern.

While the CDC has been a leading provider of developmental milestone guidelines, they do not include all categories nor ages of development in their guidelines. As both a professional and a parent, I've found that frustrating and have spent hours online, researching what is age-appropriate behavior and expectations for categories such as attention, managing upsets, screen usage, and social interactions. In this book I have compiled a variety of respected resources, from the traditional CDC guides to Stanford University, Scholastic, the U.S. Department of Health and Human Services, Brain Balance, optometrists, psychologists, and more, to save you the hours of research I've spent to better understand your kids.

Coordination Development Milestones
for Infants and Toddlers

Updated CDC guidelines:[13]

Two months:

- Holds head up when on tummy
- Moves both arms and both legs
- Opens hands briefly

Four months:
- Holds head steady without support when you are holding him
- Holds a toy when you put it in his hand
- Uses his arm to swing at toys
- Brings hands to mouth
- Pushes up onto elbows/forearms when on tummy

Six months:
- Rolls from tummy to back
- Pushes up with straight arms when on tummy
- Leans on hands to support herself when sitting

Nine months:
- Gets to a sitting position by herself
- Moves things from one hand to her other hand
- Uses fingers to "rake" food toward himself
- Sits without support

Twelve months:
- Pulls self to standing
- Walks holding on to furniture

Fifteen months:
- Takes a few steps on own

Eighteen months:
- Walks without holding on to anyone or anything
- Climbs on and off a couch or chair without help

Two years:
- Kicks a ball
- Runs
- Walks (not climbs) up a few stairs with or without help

Thirty months:
- Jumps off ground with both feet

Three years:
- Coordination to put on loose clothes such as pants or a jacket
- Uses a fork

Three to four years:[14]
- Walks backward/forward, turns and stops well

- Jumps off low steps but finds it hard to jump over objects
- Begins to ride trike and pump legs on swings
- Stands on one foot unsteadily
- Plays actively, but tires suddenly

Four years:[15]

- Catches a ball most of the time
- Can serve self food or pour water with adult supervision
- Unbuttons some buttons
- Holds crayon or pencil between fingers and thumb, not fist

Four to five years:[16]

- Skips unevenly
- Runs well
- Stands on one foot for five seconds or more
- Alternates feet when walking down stairs
- Jumps on a small trampoline
- Increased endurance in play

A key to early development is the *core postural muscles,* which provide the foundation of developing coordination. Very few parents realize the importance of the core muscles. Sometimes parents are told that their child has "low muscle tone," but they rarely grasp the full meaning and implication of that statement. Parents typically focus on the symptom that's the most prominent or most stressful. For the child who melts down or can't pay attention, the focus is on their behavior or attention. And yet, often underneath those symptoms and behaviors is a child who has weak or poor muscle tone, so they cannot develop according to the accepted milestones.

Coordination doesn't start with the ability to catch a ball while running. It starts much more simply, with the muscles—specifically the core postural muscles. These are the muscles that support the spine, provide a foundation for body movements, and support the body whether seated, standing, or running. The core trunk muscles are some of the first muscles to develop in infancy, and they help support and stabilize an infant's large head and provide the strength for future movements like rolling, sitting, and crawling.

I'm a visual learner, and when I think about the postural muscles, I envision that these muscles control the idle speed of the brain. The more revved up and fired up these muscles are, the more they rev up and fire up the brain through the RAS, so that the brain is focused, energized, and taking in information and reacting accordingly. Remember that day you spent reading on the couch and ended up sluggish and exhausted? That was because you didn't rev up and fire up the brain through muscle activation. Your RAS was idling at a low speed and produced lower levels of alertness and engagement.

So how do we apply this fascinating information to our kids, their coordination, and their development? By engaging the core postural muscles and moving! The ways to engage and move vary based on age and ability, but the purpose and goals remain the same. **Engage the muscles to engage the brain, to take in more sensory input, to understand what's happening in the world around you.**

Core postural muscles are needed for a baby to learn how to sit, crawl, and walk, providing them with the ability to explore the world around them—and to chase the family pet. Providing opportunities to engage and strengthen these muscles activates the nerves and networks in the brain that will aid in your child's movement and coordination.

Taking care of an infant while juggling other aspects of life—siblings, work, sanity, and sleep—is not easy. More and more gadgets and tools for convenience are developed each year to help entertain and engage babies, and while many of these gadgets are great, you must use them wisely.

Because I used bouncy seats, I was able to shower or make dinner when I was a first-time mom. The gentle motion, dangling toys, and noises both calmed and entertained Morgan, our oldest. There's certainly a time and a place to use a bouncy seat. However, applying what we know about the RAS and core muscles, you shouldn't use bouncy seats *all* the time. Balance seat time with tummy time. When your baby is lying in a bouncy seat, car seat, or swing, they fully relax their core postural muscles because their body is completely supported. They can kick their arms and legs and bring their hands to their face—and even their feet to their mouth—for sensory exploration, but that doesn't engage their core. Tummy time engages those muscles and puts both your baby and their brain to work! Lifting that giant bald baby head takes serious effort, engages those core postural muscles, and wakes up the brain for heightened sensory input.

Case in point: One morning a few years ago, I received a frantic text and could feel the stress vibrating through the phone.

"Help! Claire is four months old and isn't rolling over yet. Should I worry? Is this a problem? What do I do?!"

Teresa was a new mom whom I knew through Brain Balance, where she had previously worked as a coach. From her time at Brain Balance, she knew how important developmental milestones were, but since Brain Balance doesn't work with children in the infant stage, she wasn't sure what to watch for or how to help her daughter. She just knew that a missed or delayed milestone could result in larger concerns down the road and wanted to address things now rather than later.

Claire was a content and happy baby who loved to eat—an adorable baby whose fat rolls had fat rolls. As a first child with a stay-at-home mom, she didn't suffer from lack of attention. She was happiest when being held or in a bouncy seat. Tummy time, the time infants spend lying on their stomach independently, was something she tolerated in short stints, but then she'd get fussy. Like all parents trying to juggle life with an infant, the bouncy seats were a huge help when Teresa needed to make dinner, get ready for the day, or work on the computer.

Because she was a fussy baby during tummy time, Claire was held or in a seat most often. While nothing's wrong with either of those, she simply wasn't spending much time on her abdomen. Tummy time can frustrate babies because it *is* hard. They must work! And this is the very work that starts to build the core trunk muscles. Tummy time also triggers a baby's reflexes, which further develops core muscles.

Because Claire was born during the pandemic, she was probably in seats and swings more than she would have been if more friends and family had been around to help. Teresa had *less* help and support than she may have had at other times. She was the only person other than her husband who spent time with Claire, and the constant holding and rocking hardly gave Teresa a moment to herself. The bouncy seat and swing were a comfort to *both* mom and daughter. (Note: There is zero judgment in this example; being a new parent can be stressful, and a crying baby hurts you as a parent. Teresa did what worked for her and her baby.)

Right away, I knew how to advise Teresa. There are two simple strategies that can often have a quick impact on helping an infant learn to roll over.

1. Tummy time. Get on the floor with your baby. Lie on your tummy, facing them, and talk to them. Watch what happens when you do this. Not only will engaging with you distract and entertain them and help them tolerate this difficult position for longer, but holding their head up in this position will also trigger a developmental reflex. The Landau reflex is activated when your infant lifts their head in tummy time. Their little legs will also pop up in the air along with their head. Triggering this reflex will activate nearly all the extensor muscles in the back—those muscles that help you with posture and movement—and it activates the RAS. When your baby starts to get tired, their head will drop down to the floor for a quick rest, and the legs will lower and rest too. When you make another noise to capture their attention, their head and legs will pop right back up, going to work again. Stay with your baby to keep them entertained and occupied, and they'll be able to exercise longer.

2. Naked time. I know this may sound questionable, but taking off that big, bulky diaper allows your baby to kick and move their legs so much more. (Tip: lay them on a blanket or two rather than your carpet and definitely keep a towel handy.) When your baby rolls from their back to their front, it requires their hips to bend and their legs to come up and then over. A diaper can interfere with this motion and make it harder for your baby to roll.

Just two days after talking to Teresa about the power of naked baby time and extra tummy time, she sent me an adorable video. Claire was rolling over, and her parents were shouting and cheering like she'd just scored the winning goal in a game.

The asymmetrical tonic neck reflex (ATNR) is another developmental reflex that contributes in a significant way to an infant's development of coordination and utilization of the core muscles. While we maintain some types of reflexes for life (like the hammer/knee reflex), other reflexes are there only a short time to aid development and are then inhibited as the brain matures and develops control. These infant, or primitive, reflexes begin as automatic reflexes that will then morph over time into controlled and coordinated movements *by choice*.

The ATNR, sometimes called the fencer's reflex, begins to activate muscles, coordination, and timing by combining movements of several body parts in a synchronized way, impacting many different early elements of coordination. Rolling, shifting from a seated position to the belly, getting into the crawling position, and even beginning to crawl are all examples of the benefits of this reflex. Research on this reflex describes it as "fine-tuning the nervous system," allowing a change in the quality of movements.[17]

To see this reflex in action, lay your baby on their back. If you shake a rattle off to the side of their head, the baby will turn their head to look toward the noise. Turning the head to the right will then cause the baby to extend their right arm and leg, so that head, arm, and leg are all facing the same direction, toward that rattle. Then, on the opposite side, the left arm and leg will flex inward. Through this reflex, the simple movement of just turning the head will impact the movement of *all four limbs*.

The first time a baby rolls from back to front is often because of this reflex. With the entire body turning and extending to one side, while the other side curls inward, the baby's body weight and momentum will cause them to roll. While this is a happy accident the first few times, your baby will soon realize they can do it by choice, providing a smidgen of control and mobility.

Each time the reflex is triggered, muscles in the neck and all four limbs are activated, which begins to create strength for intentional movement. This also activates the corresponding regions in the brain. Over time, through repetition, the brain matures to a point of being able to override the reflex. Engaging the reflex over and over is what helps this developmental process of shifting from a reflexive response to a controlled action. An older child may hear a noise and turn to find the source of the noise. If they've outgrown this reflex, they can *choose* whether or not to reach toward the object or move in a different direction.

The ATNR impacts many factors of coordination, including aspects of crawling. Before a baby is up on all fours and can coordinate movement of all four parts in the cross-crawl pattern, they begin with an army crawl on their belly. This belly crawl involves the arm and leg on the *same side* of the body working together to drag, push, and pull that baby belly across the floor to the object of interest.

When a baby, or child of any age, does *not* mature beyond this primitive reflex, they will have *less* control over their body and the subsequent movements and coordination. For that child, moving one body part will still activate additional body parts, making control of complex movements more challenging. This lack of control can make coordinated tasks much more difficult and frustrating.

Picture a child riding their bike. They *should* be able to look over their shoulder while continuing to ride straight ahead. The child who has maintained the ATNR reflex will move in the direction their head turns. This can complicate many areas, including balance and coordination.

When a baby is held or supported in a bouncy seat or car seat, there's less opportunity to exercise this reflex, just like with core postural muscles. So while I would *never* discourage anyone from snuggling a baby, I *do* encourage being intentional about giving babies the opportunity to explore movement and coordination with *lots* of tummy time! It doesn't have to be for long periods of time. Even 5 minutes every hour that they're awake can provide lots of time for them to work those muscles and reflexes.

Mindlessly scrolling through social media one day, I paused on a video a friend posted of her baby. The caption read, "Look at Campbell, doing her thing her own way from day 1. Who needs to get their hands dirty crawling when you can cruise around this way?!"

Little Campbell was working hard to get across the room to her mom, but instead of crawling on all fours, she was scootching on her butt. Admittedly, it was some seriously impressive scootching. It was clear this was not new, as she was quite speedy.

While the video was adorable, all I could think was, *Hmm. That's not the way to build core strength and coordination.* Now, I'm not trying to say that Campbell isn't going to grow up to be amazing, but from what I do know about the brain, scootching was not engaging her reflexes, core muscles, or coordination of brain networks in the same way that crawling would. In fact, she was possibly doing this crawling alternative because of a deficit in her core muscle activation. There is no downside to engaging core muscles and primitive reflexes for your kids, and it could potentially help things such as altered crawling patterns like Campbell's.

Remember baby Claire, whose mom was worried about her lack of rolling over? After learning the importance of tummy time and core activation, she made sure Claire had tons of tummy time going forward, and Claire sat, crawled, and walked beautifully—and was on time for future milestones. All that tummy time and rolling gave her ample opportunity to trigger the ATNR, and it aided in developing more complex coordination.

Jax was another baby who was born during the pandemic to a friend of mine here in Raleigh—another parent in isolation who juggled work, older children, school, and being at home with an infant.

Because the older siblings were all at home, Jax had lots of attention. He was waited on hand and foot and loved to sit, smile, shriek, and interact with the chaos around him. But he wasn't crawling or even scootching. Jax could go from seated into the crawling position on all fours, but then he'd fall back down onto his tummy. Then he would become fussy. He could see a toy he wanted, but he couldn't get to it.

Jax's dad called one day and asked if I had any ideas about how to help.

"He's so close to crawling, and I can tell how badly he wants to. But there have been weeks of this, and he hasn't progressed. He's eleven months old. Our other kids were all crawling by now, and I feel like he should be too."

I asked his dad to take a few videos of Jax wearing only his diaper, so I could see his movements. After a few seconds of watching Jax, the complication was evident. Jax's core muscles were holding him back. When he was on all fours, he couldn't maintain the position for long. His back would droop and his baby belly would sag. The sagging belly pushed out his knees, and Jax would end up back on his tummy in frustration.

The next complication was that when he was on all fours, he used his toes to provide leverage, which worked against him when trying to crawl. His tucked toes pushed his weight forward onto his hands, and when he tried to lift a hand to crawl, he fell forward. So yes, Jax was close to being ready to crawl, but his lack of core strength and his toe position, which was a compensation for weak core strength, impeded the process.

Jax needed a little extra core strength and some guidance in keeping his feet flat while crawling (in the all-fours position, the tops of the feet should remain in contact with the floor, rather than the toes tucked under to grip). Because a baby's brain and body learn so quickly, I was confident that with a little help, Jax would be crawling in a matter of days—but this would be a two-step process.

I told his dad that he'd be spending the next few days on the floor with Jax, but if he took the time to do it, we'd most likely see some quick progress. First, I had him get Jax's attention and place a toy just out of reach, so he'd want to move to get it. Then, each time Jax shifted from seated into the crawling position, I taught Dad how to support his body. The goal was to support his tummy lightly *and* provide support on the outside of Jax's knees, to prevent his legs from spreading out wide and plopping him back down on his belly. Dad figured out how to sit with one of his feet next to Jax's knees, so he could have one hand on Jax's belly and the other hand supporting the other knee.

Once in this all-fours position, I wanted Jax to just hang out there, not trying to move forward quite yet. Babies in the all-fours position will rock back and forth as they are getting ready to crawl. Not only is this adorable, as you can see how badly they want to learn this new trick of mobility, but, as you probably guessed, it also triggers another developmental reflex—the symmetrical tonic neck reflex (STNR). Jax would not only be working his core muscles in this position, he'd also be exercising that reflex.

The STNR is another reflex that helps develop coordination. Rather than coordinating the sides of the body to work together (right arm working with right leg), it triggers the top half and bottom half of body coordination. This reflex begins with the movement of the head forward and back and the corresponding body movements that involve the arms flexing and the hips extending.[18] You can see this in action when a baby is on all fours and they move their head to look up: it triggers their hips to flex, shifting their weight back toward their heels. When they move their head to look down, the hips straighten out, shifting the body weight forward toward the hands, and the arms will bend at the elbows.

Shifting the weight forward and back helps the baby start to sense and learn how their body position impacts their ability to move. When their weight is shifted forward, if the baby tries to lift a hand to crawl, it usually results in a face plant. Shifting the weight back allows a more stable position for lifting a hand and the opposite knee in order to start propelling that little body forward successfully. As Jax's dad supported Jax in the all-fours position, he could exercise this reflex more successfully. He still wasn't crawling, but he was maintaining this position a little longer on his own.

The next step was to adjust how Jax put his feet while in this position. Dad gently held his feet so that the tops of his feet were resting in his hands, preventing those toes from curling under to grip the floor. While his dad got a sore back and knees, it was totally worth it, because Jax started crawling within a few days. Core strength and baby developmental reflexes worked their magic for the win!

Coordination Development Activities
for Infants and Toddlers

Be sure to try:
- Daily tummy time
- Tummy time propped on pillows
- Crawling through obstacle courses—over pillows, under chairs

- Crawling on uneven surfaces—the grass, the couch, a bed, a trampoline
- Jumping with two feet: up and down, over a line, from box to box in hopscotch
- Walking in a figure-eight pattern with circles on the ground
- Playing with a balance ball, lying on the ball on tummy
- Supporting your child in a seated position on an exercise ball while leaning your child from side to side for balance. Core muscles will engage to help counter and maintain balance.
- Standing on an exercise disc or a stack of pillows
- Timing play—sing songs, play clapping games, sing or talk to the rhythm of walking
- Wheelbarrowing down the hall for bedtime
- Somersaulting down the hallway for bath time

You should also:
- Minimize the use of seats. Save the seats for when you really need them!
- Give naked baby time for greater range of motion
- Guide your child in the lizard crawling exercise to exercise the ATNR: While they are lying on their tummy, turn their head to the right and have their right arm reaching up at a 90 degree angle and their right leg doing the same, so the head is facing the hand and both arm and leg are extended out and bent. Then shift to the left, so the head turns to the left, and the left arm and leg extend out, with the right arm and leg returning to the starting position. Continue to switch back and forth. In the beginning it is okay to guide your child through this exercise, helping them to turn their head and position their arms and legs. Work toward them being able to do this independently without guidance or cuing from you! To impact coordination, ideally do this exercise daily for three to twelve months.
- To exercise the STNR, have your child on their hands and knees in a cat position. Moving only the head, have your child look as far

up to the ceiling as they can, extending their head back, then help them tuck their chin to their chest, flexing the neck forward. If their body shifts forward or backward, or their arms bend while doing this exercise, gently cue them to keep their body still and solid while moving. Continue to do this exercise daily until they can move the head without that movement impacting movement in other body parts.

Elementary School Students

You may have been quite attentive to your children's motor development when they were babies or preschoolers but haven't given it another thought since they started school. Even as kids get older, what they're doing—or not doing—physically contributes to their brain development and brain function. And while coordination benchmarks are less discussed at these ages, there are still milestones for elementary-aged kids that you'll want to know.

Coordination Development Milestones
for Elementary School Students

Five years:[19]
- Can button some buttons
- Hops on one foot

Five to six years:[20]
- Walks backward quickly
- Skips and runs with agility and speed
- Incorporates motor skills into games
- Can walk a two-inch-wide balance beam easily
- Jumps over objects
- Hops well
- Jumps down several steps
- Climbs well
- Coordinates movement for swimming or biking
- Has high energy levels in play

- Rarely shows fatigue
- Finds inactivity difficult and likes active games and environments

Six to seven years:[21]

- Jumps rope
- Rides a bike
- Practices skills in order to get better

Seven to eight years:[22]

- Holds and moves across monkey bars
- Safely performs a forward roll
- Runs smoothly with opposing arms and legs and narrow foot base
- Runs around obstacles while maintaining balance
- Steps forward with leg on opposite side of throwing arm when throwing

Eight to nine years:[23]

- Shows increased coordination for throwing and catching
- Able to participate in active games with rules
- Can perform sequence motor activities, like gymnastics or shooting baskets
- Shows improved reaction time in responding to a thrown ball or oncoming vehicle
- Is more graceful with movement and abilities
- Can use tools, such as a hammer and a screwdriver

Nine years:[24]

- Becomes increasingly interested in team sports, such as soccer

Core strength and matured reflexes are just as critical in the early school years as they are in infancy, but at this age, the challenges that hold back a child's interactions and development become less obvious. Knowing what clues to watch for when it comes to core and coordination can help you know where to focus to help your child.

Your child's posture, activities, and struggles can provide insight into their skills and areas that need support. Children gravitate toward what they *can* do and are good at, and they fight, avoid, or have behavioral flare-ups around tasks that are more difficult. When it comes to posture, notice how your child sits when seated at the table and stands when in line at the grocery store. What you observe can give you a quick sense of their core strength. Sitting or standing up straight with shoulders back and head over the shoulders requires back muscle engagement. Rounded, slouched shoulders and back do not.

Keep in mind that during the pandemic years, sports and active play were reduced for kids—and there was a massive increase in technology usage that hasn't gone away even as life has resumed a more normal cadence. Technology is typically not your friend when it comes to building core strength. Not too many people sit up perfectly straight while on the computer or while zoning out in front of a video game. It's more likely that they're slouched forward with their elbows on their knees with the gaming controller in hand or sprawled back on the couch. Like babies in a bouncy seat, this doesn't engage core muscles or activate the RAS, the system that alerts the brain to be awake, focused, and alert. Building core strength that supports good posture keeps the alerting system in the brain engaged.

Parents often equate an active child with a strong child. At Brain Balance, we always check core muscle strength in kids to get a sense if they are age appropriate. More often than not, parents are surprised when I share that their child is *behind* in core strength for their age. "But he plays soccer twice a week!" or, "He never sits still. He's always running around. I know he's strong." Strong legs or arms are not indicators of core postural strength. You can be a soccer player and still have slouched posture due to poor core strength and stamina. Engaging the core muscles to support the body and movement is key for all ages to drive brain stimulation and engagement.

After observing your child's posture, take note of their coordination. How do they move? Is it smooth, fluid, and coordinated? Or is it stiff and awkward? Or different from their peers?

As a child, I personally experienced a coordination pattern that was different from my peers, and my kindergarten teacher pointed it out to me. She stopped the entire class one day as we were heading up the stairs to the school library on the second floor.

"Rebecca," she said, "you're walking up the stairs wrong. When you walk, you need to let your feet take turns." She had me come to the front of the line, and while she held my hand, she showed me—and the class—how to walk up the stairs with alternating feet.

Who knew there was a "wrong" way to walk up the stairs?! I had let my right foot lead and do all the work. Right foot up. Left foot joined. Right foot up again, and so on, never doing a cross-crawl pattern, only a one-sided pattern. Evidently, a five-year-old was too old to walk up the stairs like that. I needed to climb the stairs like a big kid and alternate my feet.

What's interesting is that I had never crawled as a baby. I was the happy baby who never developed the core strength to support my belly and eventually went from sitting to walking. Because I didn't practice either the military crawling with same-sided coordination or the traditional crawling with cross-crawl coordination, I'd missed engaging and exercising some of my developmental reflexes. As a result, I had to learn and practice what other kids did naturally. I had to learn to walk up the stairs. The gap in my coordination was a red flag that I needed extra work and support for my development. I definitely blame that gap in development for my reaction to any sports involving hand-eye coordination. I duck and cover rather than catch any ball thrown my way every time!

One day, mid-pandemic, I decided to shake up my morning routine. It was a beautiful day, so instead of driving to Starbucks for my latte, I walked. This required me to take a route through a neighborhood I rarely passed through.

As I was walking down a hill, I could see a father and son ahead of me in the street. The kid was on a bike, and Dad was behind him, hanging on. What at first appeared to be a sweet and exciting moment of childhood—learning to ride a bike—turned out to be anything but. I could see it was *not* going well. At all. Father and son started out together with the kid trying to pedal. Even with Dad jogging along the steering was wobbly, and as soon as Dad let go, the boy swerved and fell. Then he'd get up slowly and try again.

As I got closer, I could not only *see* the challenges but *hear* them too. The dad was shouting, and the child was crying. I also noticed that the boy wasn't as young as I'd first thought. He was probably eight or nine, rather than five or six—the age you'd expect a child to learn to ride a bike without training wheels. The last thing I saw before turning the corner was the boy standing with his head down and arms crossed and a dad who was also obviously frustrated.

I so badly wanted to interfere and tell them both to just *stop.* Stop yelling at the boy for failing at something he wasn't ready to do. Stop the tears that were from wounded pride as much as they were from scuffed knees and hands. Stop the process I could see was going to fail. As much as I wanted to stop and help, I knew it probably wouldn't be welcome, so I continued to get my caffeine, pondering the scene I'd just watched.

I didn't know this family, so I had no idea about the history that led up to this moment in time. For all I knew, the child had begged to try again, or maybe they'd been working on balance and coordination for months. What I knew for sure was that the boy's skills—regardless of his age—were better suited to a big wheel or bike with training wheels on that particular day.

If things aren't going well, trying the same thing over and over isn't the most efficient way to make progress for many things in life, including learning to ride a bike. Instead, break the task down into individual components and master each of those before going back to the bike.

Riding a bike requires balance, pedaling, and steering all at the same time. It's a lot to coordinate all at once. I could see the boy struggled with each of those elements. He would tip over the second his dad let go of him, so his balance wasn't there. His dad kept reminding him (by shouting) to pedal, and it was clear that it wasn't a smooth or fluid process.

If I were a betting person, I'd wager that this boy would benefit from exercising his ATNR as well as his core muscles in addition to balance and coordination. I've seen success in bike riding when the underlying functions are addressed first.

Our neighbor Andrew was a more successful example of learning to ride a bike, which was a fun surprise, since he wasn't usually the most coordinated kid when he was young. If all the neighbors were out running around and somebody got hurt, odds were good that it was Andrew.

My daughter, Morgan, is a year older than Andrew, and since she was riding a two-wheel bike, Andrew decided he should too. Knowing his clumsy reputation, his mom cringed, worried this wouldn't go well.

Luckily, Andrew, who was five at the time, was just finishing his Brain Balance program. At the beginning of the program, his core strength, coordination, balance, and timing were all one to two years behind what was age appropriate. Further, he hadn't outgrown several of his primitive reflexes, which contributed to his coordination challenges. So even though he was five, aspects of his motor coordination were closer to those of a three- or four-year-old. Putting a three- or four-year-old on a bike would *not* be successful. Understanding Andrew's coordination levels helped his mom understand why some of his movements were on the clumsy side. The good news is that by the end of his Brain Balance program, those same functions were all either at or above age appropriate, and he'd integrated most of the reflexes. Even though his mom was worried, his proficiency in the skills needed for riding a bike was there.

I left to go to the grocery store, and by the time I got back home Andrew was riding up and down our driveway on two wheels with a massive grin on his face. Because he had the balance, coordination, and timing needed to ride a bike, he learned to do it in about 20 minutes. About that same time, he began swimming without floaties and his running also took off, as did his confidence.

The three months Andrew spent at Brain Balance exercising his primitive reflexes and building core strength, coordination, timing, and other functions made a huge difference in his movements and abilities. While the neighborhood crew may still tease him about being clumsy based on his history, today he is an active middle schooler who plays soccer and baseball.

The lesson from my lack of stair climbing and Andrew's clumsy early years is that when your child's coordination doesn't align with that of their peers, it's a red flag regarding development. But it doesn't have to stay that way. When you identify the challenge and go back to some of the basics in development to coordinate brain pathways, you can propel things forward to close the gap.

Coordination Development Activities
for Elementary School Students

- ATNR and STNR support: Review activities in the infants and toddlers section and incorporate any activities your child may struggle doing, including the exercises for ATNR and STNR.
- Core muscles support: Move! Keep movement fun and playful. Talk about the positives of movement for both physical and brain health. In my opinion, it is important to make exercise a positive, not a negative, and never use it as punishment. A negative way to use exercise would be saying, "You're driving me nuts right now, go run laps around the house!" Instead, frame exercise by the benefits: "When you run/bike outside you are using your muscles to turn on your brain!"
  - Run, sprint, jump, bike, move, play, swim
  - Play catch, pickleball, frisbee in the driveway
  - Have family sit-up/push-up challenges. Record how many you can do, and each week see if you can beat last week's numbers.
  - Play games such as Twister, Simon says, hopscotch, charades, bean bag toss
  - Do yard work—push a lawn mower, pull weeds, dig dirt, rake
- Coordination support: Think about movement and form while doing an activity.
  - Run with arms and legs alternating. If the alternating pattern is smooth and natural, focus on form—moving so arms swing forward and back without any rotation. Think about foot strike and stride length.
  - Practice jumping jacks, burpees, and jumping rope; these are all great ways to work both muscles and coordination
  - Swim—pay attention to using arms and legs equally, and with good timing
  - Do agility ladder drills. YouTube has tons of great videos with fun drills. Start by using those videos for guidance, then have your kids make up their own agility patterns!

○ Change the timing of the activity. If your child is doing it fluidly, speed it up. Can your child maintain the pattern going faster? Then slow it down. Can they maintain control and coordination going slow? Slow can sometimes be harder for kids than fast.

- To make movements more complex, combine two things at a time. They can be two physical activities, or one physical and one cognitive.

  ○ Catch a ball, then catch a ball while running, or while balancing on one leg

  ○ Hop while singing a song

  ○ Skip while doing math facts

  ○ Do a coordinated activity with music—sync the movements to the beat of the music. March, bike, skip, hopscotch, throw and catch, agility ladder to the beat!

Middle School and High School Students

You probably don't picture a thirteen-year-old child and think about what they do in terms of gross motor milestones. But important motor development is still happening at this age through increased speed and intricacy.

While the major motor milestones should have been achieved by now, development at this age continues to perfect, refine, and increase in complexity with coordination. Higher-level development becomes about *control* and *inhibition*—the ability to do the right movement or action in the correct moment. And also *not* do or say something at the wrong moment. The ability to develop inhibitory control not only impacts the coordination of physical movements, but also of thoughts and actions. Control is the ability to stop a repetitive or anxious thought, or stop a movement or action.

Coordination Development Milestones for Middle School and High School Students

While there aren't formal coordination milestones for this age group, there are recommendations for physical activities that adolescents should have the strength and endurance to achieve. The Presidential Youth Fitness Program standards provide goals for physical fitness that were designed to be implemented in schools to motivate and encourage physical fitness and overall wellness.[25] These guidelines stress the importance of regular physical activity for many aspects of health, including cardiovascular wellness as well as mental health and cognition. The guidelines state, "Compared to those who are inactive, physically active youth have higher levels of cardiorespiratory fitness and stronger muscles. They also typically have lower body fat and stronger bones. Physical activity also has brain health benefits for school-aged children, including improved cognition and reduced symptoms of depression. **Evidence indicates that both acute bouts and regular moderate-to-vigorous physical activity improve the cognitive functions of memory, executive function, processing speed, attention, and academic performance for these children.**"[26]

The Presidential Youth Fitness Program recommendations below were last updated in 2021.[27]

- Adolescents are recommended to have 60 minutes per day of moderate to vigorous aerobic physical activity
- As part of the daily 60 minutes of physical activity, at least three days a week should include muscle strengthening activities
- As part of the daily 60 minutes of physical activity, at least three days a week should include bone strengthening activities. Healthcarefix .com describes bone strengthening exercises as those that have been shown to increase bone density through weight-bearing and muscle strengthening exercises.[28] Examples of these exercises include activities such as brisk walking, running, jumping, yoga, and weight lifting.

In the teen years and beyond, coordination should also involve the ability to incorporate several tasks at once. Dribbling a basketball while running down the court or skating on ice while stick handling a puck are two examples in sports that demonstrate this ability for layered complexity of coordination.

Basic coordination expectations include:[29]

- Your child can actively partake in sports

- They have good balance and coordination in relation to a variety of tasks
- They have found and enjoy certain active hobbies

The ability to develop better control and inhibition is still aided by core postural muscles at this age. Engaging in activities that involve precise timing and decision making contributes to the control and inhibition needed to succeed in life. There are great ways to exercise and improve these functions in the brain that not only enhance the accuracy of athletic and coordinated movements but translate into control and inhibition capabilities in other areas of life too. (What teen wouldn't benefit from better timing, decision making, and impulse control?)

If you're not sure how core muscles impact your teen and their mood or hobbies, take a moment to consider. Whether they're shooting a goal in hockey, dancing for a solo competition, playing the piano, or even playing some video games, their core muscles are involved—either by providing a stable base for movement or by keeping the brain alert and engaged. Remember that postural muscles help in increasing focus, behavior, mood, and energy. If the core muscles are weak, it results in more sluggish execution of movement and actions.

In fact, due to the natural changes that begin to occur at this age, it becomes even more important to be *intentional* about finding ways to engage and work the muscles for our teenagers. When kids were younger, they naturally moved to drive development and explore the world, constantly running, playing, and climbing. Can you imagine how fit we'd be as adults if we continued to move that much? Then puberty kicks in, along with all that goes with it—suddenly kids are experiencing mood changes, seeking privacy, and sleeping as late as possible or is tolerated by parents. Teens' version of play is different. Hanging out with friends may involve sitting around and staring at their phones or going to a movie rather than running around the neighborhood like they used to do.

Add to that the physical changes that puberty brings and the upheaval from the pandemic years, when there was less movement, more stress, and more technology. Obesity rates increased at all ages during this time because these changes also impacted our eating and sleeping patterns. The result is that millions of teens are not moving their bodies enough or are not moving in ways that help their brains, moods, and energy.

Muscles are "use it or lose it." Month after month of minimal movement results in a sluggish body and brain.

I witnessed an example of muscles firing up the brain and mood firsthand with friends during the pandemic one summer. We were spending a day on the lake water skiing with friends.

Nate was driving the boat, and before his son, Ely, took his turn skiing, he turned to me and whispered, "Watch this."

"Huh?" I responded.

Leaning over, Nate said, "Watch Ely when he gets back into the boat. Exercise gives the kid a blast of energy."

Sure enough, Ely, who'd been quiet on the boat, was on fire when he got back from skiing. He'd had a great run (the kid is an amazing slalom skier) and was excited to dissect it with his dad and cheer on the next skier. The difference in his demeanor before and after his run was like night and day. It was astounding. I started observing the other kids, and it wasn't only Ely who crawled back into the boat energized. As for me, I too was energized and grinning from ear to ear after my turn, although I was barely able to stand.

While we need our core muscles to support our body and engage the brain, successful coordination is also completely dependent on timing. A great baseball swing that's a split-second behind the pitch results in a strike, not a home run. In swimming, all four limbs are moving, but if they don't move in sync, you get a lot of splashing but not a lot of swimming.

Timing impacts more aspects of life than you realize. In fact, your abilities in so many areas—pronouncing a word, telling a story, writing an essay, playing sports—all come down to timing. If the timing is off, the word is mispronounced or the story doesn't make sense. Timing with complex synchronization requires multiple aspects of the brain to come online together to execute the task. By working to improve your child's coordination, you're also working to improve their brain's ability to execute on timing.

I frequently get questions and comments from parents regarding timing and reaction time related to video games. Their comments are usually along the lines of, "I see how fast my kids can navigate the game and controller, and I can barely keep up when watching, so why do they still struggle with homework, tests, sports, and behavior when they're so good with video games?"

The answer is simple. Real life and video games aren't the same. When playing a video game, the child is laser-focused on the task at hand, and all they need to coordinate is what they see and how their thumbs move, versus everything they need to synchronize and coordinate when playing a sport.

Picture lacrosse. It involves holding the stick, cradling the ball, running, dodging, and pivoting while keeping your eye on the ball and knowing the play and how your teammates are moving. There is a lot happening all at once. There are massive skills and talent involved in gaming, but you can't expect those skills to translate into the physical realm.

The ultimate skill to maximizing your physical coordination is the ability to *decide* when it's the right time to do the thing you're doing. It's your ability to override an instinct—that is, impulse control. It's what we call *inhibition*—having the right action in the right moment.

Impulse control means you don't swing at every pitch in baseball. You exercise the ability to choose when to react and when to hold back. It means you don't slam your stick on the ice when you miss a shot in hockey. And you don't fall off the balance beam when you start to wobble. Impulse control means working on your swimming stroke when you'd rather default to bad habits that slow you down.

In the science world, these tasks are known as *go-no-go* tasks. These are tasks where in a split-second you need to make a decision to go—or not. Picture the game red light, green light you played as a child. If you were "it," when you said "green light" everyone ran toward you. Then you'd call out "red light," and they'd have to slam on the brakes and freeze. If you saw someone moving after calling red light, you would call their name, and they were out of the game.

The best athletes excel at control, and they continue to work at it to stay at the top of their game. You may be thinking to yourself, *My goal isn't for my kid to be a top athlete, or to be an athlete at all, so why is this relevant?* When the brain can successfully synchronize coordination, timing, and control to execute a physical task, it carries over into other areas of life as well—areas like decision making and impulse control also involve connecting multiple pathways simultaneously. And guess what? You can set up an agility ladder at home and do exercises and drills to work on timing and impulse control much easier than you can practice other moments in life when impulse control is needed.

If you see an increase in negative moods and behaviors in your children during and after times when they have had little to no physical activity, this is important to note. We know a tired and sluggish brain has less ability to pay attention, coordinate a response, and control that response. Kids who spend less time moving, and more time on technology, often have more issues with mood, emotions, and behaviors than kids who remain more consistently active.[30] (There's a reason exercise is so important when facing mental health challenges such as depression.)

So, whether or not your child is an athlete, your child's focus, energy, mood, and impulse control will benefit from engaging postural core muscles and working on physical coordination, timing, and impulse control. In fact, as a parent, you'll benefit from working on these things with your child. I know I do.

Coordination Development Activities for Middle School and High School Students

- Review the activities in the infants and toddlers and elementary school students sections and incorporate any activities your child may struggle doing.
- Find movement that your child likes even if they are not a "sporty" kid. It doesn't have to be a team sport to be an active activity. Yoga, Pilates, running, biking, rollerblading, paddle boarding, rock climbing, canoeing, skateboarding, and surfing are all great ways to exercise.
- Use an app to guide daily exercises for building core strength, and work it into a daily routine with as little as 5–15 minutes to begin with, and gradually increasing over time.

- At this age social interactions become more important—sign up for group activities and classes. Think beyond team sports—Girls on the Run is a nonprofit group that focuses on empowerment, and there are lots of other running clubs, as well as hiking groups, rock climbing teams, kayaking groups, and mountain biking clubs.

- Choose a category such as hikes, waterfalls, mountain bike trails, soda shops, or frisbee golf courses and then explore your area to visit as many of those locations as you can. Work together with your child to brainstorm fun ideas or categories to spend time exploring.

- Sign up with friends or as a family for a race or an event like the Color Run, a 5k run where you get doused in colorful powder.

Signs That Indicate Improvement

You'll know you're on the right track for improving coordination and timing when you first begin to see an increase in your child's core strength. Look for improved posture and mobility or an increase in endurance. You might start to notice less complaining when it comes to physical activities and stamina. As your child's strength, coordination, and timing begin to synchronize more effectively, you'll see your child naturally gravitate toward activities that are active and require coordination, like riding their bike, dribbling a basketball in the driveway, or playing catch. You may notice their movements are more smooth when walking, running, and jumping—and if not, keep at it until you do. Highly perceptive parents will notice that an improvement in timing and physical coordination correlates with improved timing in other areas like speech, conversations, thought, and actions.

2

....

SENSORY DEVELOPMENT

The human experience is a rich and varied one thanks in large part to the development of our senses. The joy of a beautiful sunset, a great song, a delicious meal, and even the feelings of love and connection with friends and family are provided to us through the intricacy of our sensory system. This system creates the opportunity for awareness of and interactions with the world around us, providing us with the ability to learn and guiding our behaviors and interactions. From the foods we choose to eat, to the conversations we have with friends, to the split-second decisions we make, our senses provide us with the information upon which we act or react.

The more research uncovers about the sensory system, the more we understand how critical these systems are to our overall well-being. In fact, a recent study shared evidence that sensory inputs have an impact on the development of our emotional circuitry—the pathways in the brain that control our emotions and responses.[1] Specifically, the primary sensory pathways that process light, sound, and touch, when paired with memory circuitry, were found to be instructive in the maturation of emotional responses.

Note to Parents

Our sensory system can provide us with many happy experiences, but this same system can also generate big feelings of stress, anxiety, and upset. There is nothing more stressful to a parent than when big emotions turn into an utter meltdown for their child. The tantrum of the toddler, the stomping feet and slamming doors of the elementary-aged child, or the shutdown or explosive anger of a teenager are all examples. While it is easy to focus on the upsetting behavior from your child, what often is missed is the sensory experience that may have contributed to pushing your child over the edge of what they can tolerate and process, or disrupted their ability to pay attention and regulate their behaviors.

You're not alone if you've noticed your kids struggling with feelings of stress or anxiety. Or with staying focused to complete a chore or homework task. Maybe some days your child is able to tolerate the noise and chaos of a busy household, and other times this same noise from siblings drives them nuts or pushes them to act out. Or you may find yourself walking on eggshells, not knowing if or when your child may melt down. Each one of these challenges can be related to the brain's capacity to process sensory input.

Sensory overload can be hard for a parent to identify and difficult for a child to understand or verbalize. Disruptions in attention and learning related to sensory experiences can also be difficult to identify but can impact learning both socially and academically. The goal for this chapter is to learn more about how the senses impact the brain, behaviors, and cognition and what you can do to help drive maturity in the sensory system.

When you understand how the brain responds to sensory information, it can provide you with better tools and approaches to support your kids—and even add to your understanding of yourself. When you know how sensory information is used to orient us, provide comfort, and support learning and development, you'll gain an appreciation of why your kids' moods and behaviors are directly impacted by their sensory experiences and environment.

Pandemic Lessons

During the pandemic, our sensory exposure decreased dramatically. We spent more time at home, interacted with fewer people, and had limited new experiences compared to pre-pandemic times. The result of the pandemic lockdown's massive disruptions to daily life was that a significant amount of our sensory exposure was curtailed. We, by necessity, limited our brains to the sensory experiences in our own homes and neighborhoods. This meant we all experienced very similar sensory input day after day after day—our own version of the movie *Groundhog Day.*

After a prolonged period of reduced exposure, readjusting to life with more sights, sounds, and experiences was overwhelming for many. Adults found themselves feeling drained, overwhelmed, or irritable. Kids would present with crankiness, as well as fatigue, meltdowns, anxiety, or difficulty focusing.

While sensory overload can happen to anyone, the pandemic's period of sensory deprivation highlighted the impact our senses have on so much of our life's experiences.

Beyond repetition and boredom, the sensory void had a concerning impact on many aspects of development. **Sensory processing is the basis of our cognitive, social, physical, and emotional skills.** Wikipedia, while not always the best source of information, provides a definition of *cognition* that I love: "the mental action or process of acquiring knowledge and understanding through thought, experiences, and the senses."[2] In short, we learn through our senses.

Human sensory systems and interpretations are critical to development. When our sensory exposure was limited, the stimulation and challenges that help support learning and development were significantly reduced, resulting in dysregulation. And this happened to an entire cohort of kids (and adults).

To counter the disruption of sensory dysregulation, we need to engage the brain repeatedly and in a variety of ways. The good news is that we can address these deficits to help get our kids back on track and thriving. And we now have a better understanding of the importance of sensory stimulation to support development in all kids as a result of this period of time. According to Senaptec, a company that offers cognitive assessments and training for athletes, nearly 80% of our brain is dedicated to processing sensory input. Any disruptions or differences in how we absorb this information can impact everything from attention and behaviors to anxiety, mood, and learning.

While sensory challenges that impact learning, mood, and emotions are concerning, research shows change can occur. Research I was involved in at Brain Balance demonstrates how doing specific exercises and activities to engage the senses and body, considered multi-modal training, can improve cognitive performance in kids, specifically those who struggle with aspects of development and attention.[3] The largest impact was found to be on measures of concentration, memory, logic, and reasoning—all key areas influenced by our sensory systems and needed to succeed in the classroom and beyond.

Our sensory system includes the obvious categories of sight, hearing, smell, taste, and touch. But there are additional sensory systems that provide critical information regarding our body position and movements through our proprioception and vestibular systems, as well as our awareness of ourselves and how we are feeling through the sense of interoception. Through these combined sensory systems, and without exerting any intentional effort, you glean a great deal of information about the environment and your body.

Science Alert

The reticular activating system we discussed in chapter 1 controls how much sensory information our brain is allowing in to process at any given time. This information in turn guides our behaviors. When an experience is new, your actions and reactions are not yet automatic, so the RAS lets more sensory information through. Because the brain has not yet determined which information is pertinent, all information is provided. Once you have experienced something over and over, and your responses become automatic, the RAS filters the sensory input so you are only receiving what is necessary in order to react.[4] Think about the first time you navigated an airport. You got off the plane and looked around, trying to figure out where to go to retrieve your luggage and find the location to get a ride to your destination. You noticed the noise of the airport and the many people milling around, and you had to read all the signs telling you where to go. You probably felt a little stressed or anxious during this time of navigating an unknown location. After flying many times through the same airport, you step off the plane with complete ease and very little thought or stress and navigate through the airport to grab your belongings while scrolling through your phone. You aren't bothered by the noise and barely notice all the people standing around or the signs guiding you to baggage claim. This is an example of the RAS muting information to your brain since you already know what is needed to complete this task. You get to conserve the energy it would have taken to process the abundance of sensory information of a new experience. In both scenarios you reach the same destination, but in the first, stressful situation, far more energy was burned to process the bombardment of sensory input. You arrived at your destination more tired and stressed.

Understanding the RAS may also explain why trauma can create heightened sensory processing and stress going forward. It is not uncommon for people to experience sensory processing issues after traumatic events.[5] For safety and protection, when the brain perceives an event as traumatic, the brain will go on high alert to make sure no critical information is missed. It will be listening for every sound, scanning the environment, tensing your muscles, and accelerating your heart rate. This state means the brain is taking in and processing a lot of information and burning through a great deal of resources, which will leave the individual feeling negative, stressed, and less in control of their emotions and reactions.

Repeated experiences create automation in the behavioral responses, which conserves energy in the brain. The brain doesn't need to process as much information nor make as many decisions. The first time your child experiences something new will be more taxing on their energy and emotions as the brain will need to filter through all the sensory information. But then experiencing something repeatedly will begin to create automation and familiarity, allowing the brain to filter out the extra information so your child's brain is focusing on only the important sensory input coming through. **Finding opportunities to create a variety of sensory experiences for your kids, then repeating those experiences, can contribute to greater efficiency and ease in situations loaded with sensory stimuli and can create learning for the brain.**

To understand how your senses provide information, try this simple experiment with me. After reading this paragraph, close your eyes and think about everything you can describe about yourself and your current environment. Consider each of your senses and what information that sense provides you.

What I notice is that I'm sitting on a comfy, overstuffed chair in my office. My lower back is a little stiff from sitting hunched over my laptop for too long. My office is warm and stuffy. I can feel the sun shining in through the window, and I hear the birds chirping outside, which tells me it's a beautiful spring day. My kids are home, but I don't hear them, so I'm not worried about how they're doing in this moment. (Although, thinking about it more, quiet doesn't always mean it's good.) I can smell the grapefruit candle I lit and can hear the puppy breathing deeply as he sleeps on his bed near my feet. I'm relaxed, a little hungry, and I'm aware that my focus is starting to wane as my thoughts are jumping all over the place right now. This indicates that I'm overdue for a snack and movement break.

Opening my eyes, I can confirm the information I understood while my eyes were closed. My senses let me know that right now my environment is safe, warm, and quiet, which allows me to feel calm, relaxed, and focused.

That feeling of calm and relaxation could change in an instant—also perceived through my senses. If I heard a loud crash and a scream from upstairs, my brain would kick into high alert, and I'd be stressed until I knew my family was okay. My senses would tell me it was time to jump into action to investigate the crash and the scream.

Now consider that same experiment, but take out one of your senses.

If you closed your eyes and were wearing noise-canceling headphones, you'd have less information to contribute to your understanding of your environment. If I couldn't hear the puppy sleeping, I might worry about what disaster he was currently creating, and I'd also wonder if the kids were calling for help or if they needed me. If I couldn't hear the birds singing outside, I wouldn't have as much information about the day and the weather.

Changing your sensory perception can alter how you feel, what knowledge you have about your environment, and your level of alertness, attention, anxiety, and fatigue.

Imagine how you'd feel trying to cross a busy road while wearing a blindfold and ear plugs. You couldn't hear or see the traffic, so you'd most likely freeze and wouldn't want to cross the street. Or if you could see and hear, but the cars were much louder than normal, you might feel like the cars were moving faster or were coming right at you. These are extreme examples, but they show how muted or amplified senses can change your interpretation of events and even increase levels of stress and anxiety.

Life and experience allow us to learn more about the information our senses provide, so over time, we become more aware and more confident in the information and nuances we detect. As our sensory processing improves, we filter out more of the unnecessary information (thanks to the RAS) and can process more information faster, resulting in more accuracy and confidence in what we perceive.

Our senses provide information, then we correlate that info with our frame of reference. This is how we reinforce something we already know or learn something new. Our senses provide us with information that we can use in the future to keep calm and be aware of what is happening around us (think of the study that demonstrated how sensory input paired with memory impacted emotional responses and circuitry in the brain).

For people who process sensory input differently—as too strong or too weak—their perceptions can *increase* rather than *decrease* their levels of stress and anxiety. They can't fully trust their senses. Rather than being grounded by sensory input, it can make them feel unsettled or unsure of their environment, and it can impact their social and learning interactions.

Altered or dysregulated sensory input can also cause them to focus on the wrong information. For example, a rock in your shoe will capture your attention and annoy you, pulling your attention from the beautiful view on your hike. For people who experience heightened input, something as simple as a seam on their sock or a tag on their pants could be the equivalent of a pebble in the shoe for you and me.

If your child experiences dysregulation or immaturity in their senses, especially in sight and sound, sitting in the classroom may feel like trying to cross a busy street blindfolded. They may struggle to keep up and constantly feel that they are missing key information. They may not trust what they do hear and see, resulting in needing instructions and information repeated over and over. With age-appropriate development, kids perceive auditory information with greater consistency. This means that they will be more accurate in what they perceive more often. With auditory processing maturity there is also an improvement in being able to direct their attention, to focus on what they want to hear while blocking out distractions.[6]

Dysregulation in sensory processing can present in many ways, including confusion and stress:

- Did I hear the teacher's instructions correctly so I can take the right notes to prepare for the test? I'm unsure, so I'm stressed about the upcoming test.

- My friend just said something and laughed. Is he laughing *at* me or *with* me? Now I don't know if this interaction is friendly or if he's making fun of me.
- I was walking down the hall and a kid bumped into me. To me, that bump felt BIG. So, was that a bump or a shove? Now I'm mad, and I want to react or retaliate.
- I read the instructions for the test, but now I'm questioning what I thought I read. Did I miss a step?

Kids who don't accurately interpret sensory information can experience disrupted or misinterpreted interactions, which can leave them feeling confused and angry. It may even appear that they're lying when their experience is different from someone else's experience of the same event.

Your sensory system can also impact your mood and energy. To understand this aspect of sensory processing, think about something that seems easy yet can leave you feeling tired or even irritable. For me, after a few hours at the mall, I feel worn down, even though all I did was walk slowly from store to store. While a trip to the mall may not sound tiring, it can be exhausting to the brain. Why does meandering for hours wear you out and bring out challenging behaviors in your kids? The answer has a lot to do with the amount of sensory input your brain needs to process and the resources your brain has available as support.

Consider all the sensory input at the mall. Visually, there's fluorescent lighting, people, stores, and all the merchandise. Auditory stimulation comes from the music in the stores and the conversations happening around you. You notice touch and temperature when people bump into you if it's crowded, or you may feel warm if you're wearing your winter coat inside. Even the weight and heft of your shopping bags provide sensory input. And the smells! There are strong scents of Cinnabon, the lotions and potions at Bath and Body Works and perfume counters, as well as the other people. If sensory input were a volume dial on the radio, going to the mall would be like turning that dial to full blast.

The brain requires fuel and energy to process the information it continually takes in, and the brain is constantly taking in *a lot* of information while you're awake. The constant stream of information gives your brain critical information about where you are, what's happening around you, whether you're safe, and if you need to move or do something different to stay safe. The brain even processes some sensory information while you're asleep, but at a much lower rate. The more sensory input you receive, the more fuel and energy your brain uses to process and react to the input.

Your brain doesn't have an unlimited supply of energy and fuel, and when it runs low or runs out, the result isn't pretty at any age. Picture how you feel when you're hangry. That's the point when you are so hungry you can't think, you can't make a decision, and you're crabby. You need food NOW. Your brain has run out of energy, and you've been zapped of the ability to use the parts that help you think, plan, and control your behaviors and reactions.

Contrast time spent at the mall with time being at home. Your house still has sensory stimulation, but it's far less than at a mall. And it's things you're more familiar with—the barking dog, the kids playing, and the smell of dinner cooking. Your brain doesn't process this info on high alert and try to determine what is happening or whether you're safe. Your actions around home are familiar and automated, allowing the brain to filter out information that is present but deemed unnecessary by your brain. You're relaxed and comfortable in a familiar environment, so your brain is also more relaxed, which requires less energy and fewer resources to process. You feel less drained after spending hours at home than you do when you're in a sensory-rich and less familiar environment.

It's easy to assume that we all experience sensory information the same way, but that's not true. In fact, studies report as many as one in six kids may have a sensory processing disorder, a condition where the brain has trouble receiving and responding to information that comes in through the senses.[7] Adults can struggle with sensory dysregulation as well. It's also important to note you don't need a diagnosis for your overloaded senses to impact your mood and interactions. Kids who experience an amplified sensory experience can become stressed and anxious in loud or chaotic environments, as their brain perceives the sights, sounds, and smells as larger than what others may experience. This heavy load of sensory input requires a great deal of energy from the brain to process. When the energy needed to process runs out, an escalation in challenging behaviors will result. Irritability, shutdown, meltdown, and less control of mood and emotions will happen when the brain no longer has the resources needed to support the inflow of information. As a parent it is easy to then discipline the behavior—the impulsive reaction, the petulant tone or action—when the reality is a child who doesn't have the resources needed to process their current experience.

It's helpful to understand that enhancing and furthering development can have a positive impact on improving sensory processing. "Sensory dysregulation tends to get better with neurological maturation," notes Allison Kawa, PsyD, a Los Angeles child psychologist.[8]

Take a look at the developmental stages below, even if your child has already passed this age, in case they missed any key steps or milestones. Highlight any missed milestones so that when you build your weekly engagement calendar, you'll be sure to include important underlying categories.

Infants and Toddlers

Life as an infant and toddler is all about sensory exploration and play since everything is new, exciting, and also exhausting. Constant learning is happening through the sensory system, whether they are experimenting with what they can control through babbling and screeching or feel through chewing on their own hand or a soft toy.

Sensory Development Milestones for Infants and Toddlers

Zero to three months:[9]
- Constantly receives information through all their senses. This information is used to learn and develop the brain.
- Turns head toward breast or bottle to be fed and away from bright light—a reaction to the information they are perceiving through the visual system
- Anticipates feeding and will orient to the smell of their caregiver/milk
- Turns to sound of sibling or pet
- Interested in faces

- Cries when uncomfortable (interoception, the ability to be aware of and interpret internal sensations and feelings—hungry, tired, in need of diaper change)
- Attempts to reach a toy above their chest—visual input to see something that captures interest and attention and then directs behavior
- Visually tracks a moving object from side to side when lying on their back
- Able to be soothed with rocking, touch, gentle sounds

Four to six months:[10]

- Can use both sides of the body together
- Uses slow movements for calming and more vigorous movements for play
- Sways back and forth
- Experiments more with force
- Claps, pets, pulls on a blanket
- Soothed by soft, cozy sensations like blankets, clothes, toys
- Starts to show interest in how foods that others are eating smell and look
- Notices toys that make sounds
- Not upset by everyday sounds

Seven to nine months:[11]

- Tries to reach, lean, throw toys
- Able to stretch, reach, and lean in many directions
- Enjoys a variety of movements like bouncing up and down, rocking back and forth
- Experiments with amount of force needed to pick up or put down an object
- Focuses on objects near and far
- Investigates shapes, sizes, and textures of toys, objects, and surroundings
- Observes environment from a variety of positions—on back, on tummy, seated, crawling, standing with assistance

- Uses hands and mouth to explore objects and toys
- Starts to look at and reach for food that is nearby
- Begins to form associations with familiar smells and tastes
- Can distinguish between familiar and unfamiliar voices
- Craves chew toys

Ten to twelve months:[12]

- Enjoys more energetic activities like playing horsey and bouncing up and down
- Puts arms over and under new spaces and objects and crawls under a table or over a cushion
- Crawls toward or away from sounds heard from a distance
- Crawls toward or away from objects seen in the distance
- Enjoys listening to songs
- Explores toys with hands, fingers, and mouth

Thirteen to eighteen months:[13]

- Eats an increasing variety of foods
- Identifies a larger variety of sounds and words
- Identifies themselves in a mirror
- Begins to be able to do more complex movements, such as climbing up stairs
- Has better control of speed of movements and can speed up or slow down as needed

As we've discussed, much of our children's sensory exposure came to a screeching halt in 2020. And while we can't change the past, we can learn from it, understanding that the disruption in sensory exposure played a part in increases in challenges with attention, mood, regulating emotions, behavior, and learning. Knowing how important our sensory system is to learning and interactions can allow us to maintain a heightened focus on supporting sensory development in our kids going forward.

Remember that huge amounts of brain pathways and resources are dedicated to our sensory systems, and when we were deprived of this exposure, we eliminated the learning and growth in kids for the systems that ground and orient us in the world.

For infants and toddlers, providing educational sensory experiences can be as simple as being mindful of the experiences you encounter in your daily life—and adding some variety into your week as well. Our little ones have spent most of their first two years of life at home, and they'll be thrilled and stimulated by anything that's new and different. And it doesn't need to be exotic to be engaging.

While errands feel like a hassle to us, they provide new and interesting experiences for our kids. Don't overlook the stimulation and learning that can take place at the grocery store or pet store. Start with a 20-minute outing to the grocery store, which provides a rich sensory experience. Even if your child has gone to the store with you many times, next time, go with a purpose and a plan for sensory enrichment—as well as to pick up the items on your list for dinner.

Pick a time when you're not in a hurry, and your child is well rested and fed. Then take your time, walk the aisles, and experience the senses together. Touch the cold on the container of ice cream, feel the texture of a cucumber and let your child hold it while you shop, shake a box of cereal, smell the flowers when you walk by. Engage all the senses and talk about what you're experiencing as you're doing it. The grocery store offers colors, textures, temperatures, smells, and sometimes even tastes. On your next trip, you can revisit some of the same foods and reinforce what you learned last time. Cucumbers are green, tomatoes are red, fresh basil smells delicious, and ice cream is cold.

Developing cognition requires that you engage the senses to create experiences. It also requires repetition. You can create short but fun routines to enjoy with your child that might make grocery shopping a more pleasurable experience for both of you.

If you're like me these days, I do as much as I possibly can online to save time, but shopping online or ordering food to be delivered eliminates the sensory experience. Work to find balance in life so on occasion you can bring your child along on a sensory outing to the local coffee shop or grocery store, where they are surrounded by a variety of aromas, sights, and sounds. Everywhere you go can provide sensory experiences when you start paying attention.

Remember the story I told you about the photographer who took portraits of one-year-olds? That real-life example taught me that our COVID-era babies are not as comfortable around new people and places compared to those born in pre-COVID times. They haven't had the same exposure to the variety of new and different people as babies had in the past. Keeping this in mind for our infants will help us provide them with a rich sensory environment in which to learn and build comfort and confidence through their senses.

Another lockdown result we all experienced was a decrease in the amount of in-person interactions and an increase in online interactions. While technology provided us welcome ways to connect with friends and family, it's not the same kind of sensory experience.

Every new person your child encounters is a sensory experience. Everyone has a unique look, smell, voice, laugh, and language. The experience of the smells, sounds, and textures of people simply cannot be translated through technology. So, if your extended family is far away, or your neighborhood is not filled with kids of all ages and families, find people outside your family unit that you can connect with to expand your child's social interactions and build their social sensory experiences.

Being exposed to different ages, languages, and races builds your child's world awareness and helps prepare them for school, where they'll share a classroom and building with many different people. Exposure to new people helps build their comfort and confidence now, so they aren't afraid of things that are new and different.

Quinn was a typical COVID-era baby—a first child for a couple in California in April 2020. Quinn's paternal grandparents lived nearby, and partway into the COVID isolation, the families figured out how to quarantine together so they could visit in person. Quinn's moms were both working from home, and they had a young nanny come to the house to care for him. With five adults in Quinn's world, it was full of consistent love and care.

Quinn's other grandparents and aunts, uncles, and cousins had seen numerous photos and videos over the eighteen-month quarantine, and in fall 2021, the family was ready for an in-person visit. Everyone was beyond excited to meet the new baby, who was now walking and talking. His maternal grandparents found a huge cabin to rent for the week, and multiple families converged at this peaceful cabin in the woods.

While the visit was wonderful in so many ways, afterward the couple shared how frustrated they'd been with Quinn's behavior. The normally happy baby, who'd always maintained a great sleep and nap schedule, was incredibly fussy throughout the week. He threw more fits and tantrums than ever. He was uncooperative when he ate and was needy and clung to his moms all week. While the extended family understood that a different schedule and routine was hard for an eighteen-month-old, Quinn's parents felt like the family didn't get to see all his wonderful aspects.

After hearing about the family vacation, I started to process what had happened. Quinn's home life was a lovely and quiet one. Two parents, a nanny, and a cat don't create as much noise and mayhem as a huge cabin filled with cousins, aunts, and uncles. Quinn had a week of absolute sensory overload. How could that week have gone well?

As much as I love time with my entire family, a week with all of us in one place would be overload for me (and my husband for sure). Going for a run in the morning and taking time on my own to read in the afternoon are things I know to do to help regulate my sensory experience and prevent me from becoming tired and irritable. As an adult, I still need to adapt to my environment. Very young children don't have that same level of awareness and ability to adapt and self-regulate, so we need to do it for them.

For his entire life, Quinn had only slept in his crib or napped in a pack 'n play at his grandparents' house—a home even quieter than his own. He'd seen and played with some neighbor kids outside but had never spent several days with older kids in his face who handed him toys, played pat-a-cake, and sang to him. Mealtime was normally a quiet time with his nanny or parents.

The cabin experience was the exact opposite. Mealtime consisted of fifteen people—eight adults and seven kids—who loaded up their plates and sat around the table eating, laughing, and talking over one another. Can you imagine how interesting and distracting this would be for a child who'd never sat at a large table with so many people? Quinn was too distracted to eat, which meant his brain and body didn't get the additional fuel they needed to help him process this bombardment of sensory input.

Not to mention all the additional sensory stimulation Quinn experienced all day: exploring a new house, playing outside near a creek and through the woods, and being surrounded by many new people, all wanting to spend time with him. He was overwhelmed and over-stimulated, and he didn't have the resources to process it all.

Babies learn through senses and repetition. Putting things in their mouths—including their own hands—is part of this process. It's how they learn self versus non-self. If the baby bites down on a toy, they don't feel it. When they bite down on their own hand and it hurts, they quickly learn that the hand belongs to them, and too much pressure isn't good.

Some areas of our bodies have more sensory receptors than others, which allows us to be aware of more subtle information from specific regions. For example, both the hands and the mouth have many more receptors than the elbows or shins. In fact, each hand has over 100,000 nerves and over 3,000 touch receptors in each fingertip.[14] Your mouth is similar, with a higher concentration of touch receptors in your lips and tongue.[15]

Daily life can provide so many sensory experiences a child can engage in with their hands and mouth. Imagine you run to the coffee shop for a muffin, swing by the park to play, go home for nap time, then over to a friend's house for a playdate. Consider all the touch opportunities for the hands and mouth: the texture of the muffin, the smooth slide and the wet sand at the park, and the pile of new and different toys at the friend's house. All new textures to play with and explore and learn.

To be clear, I'm *not* suggesting you allow your child to eat the wet sand and lick their friend's toys. I *am* suggesting that you find safe ways for your child to have a variety of textures and objects of differing levels of soft, hard, smooth, and firm to explore. And to even put these things up to their mouth to explore. This will help their brain begin to catalogue new information. A teddy bear's foot is squishy and hairy and feels fuzzy in the mouth. A board book is smooth and hard to bite into. As goofy as this sounds, it provides your child important information, contributing to their learning.

Parks, nature, and the great outdoors provide free and varied sensory exposure and experiences: the wind ruffling your hair, the warm sun on your face, the smell of wet sand, the feel of the slide, the noises of other kids and parents, the experience of running and laughing. There is so much brain engagement from so many different regions, all firing in concert to process all the information. It's a comprehensive sensory experience, and it's no wonder kids nap so well after time outside or at the park.

This needs to happen as much as possible now for all kids, big and small, especially as we navigate the ever-increasing use of technology and its impact on our own sensory stimuli and sanity. We need to learn from the lessons of the sensory vacuum we created and instead fill that space with sensory-rich experiences.

Sensory Development Activities for Infants and Toddlers

Ways to engage each sense

Remember, it doesn't need to be fancy or elaborate for it to be a new and beneficial sensory experience for your little one. Kids love routine, so create routines and habits around the senses that include some of their favorite activities in addition to finding something new and different to experience each day or on the weekend.

Sight
- Get out of the house.
- Visit parks, trails, neighborhoods, the grocery store, a department store, a pet store (go look at the guinea pigs, birds, fish, and kittens), the library, bookstore, local nature center, and Grandma's house.
- Think about a variety of nature sights to experience: streams, ponds, lakes, the ocean, fields, hills, mountains, sidewalks, wood chip paths, dirt paths, grass, and turf.
- Hold your child so they can see the same things from a different angle. In your backyard, they can peek over the fence; in the house, they can see higher shelves or the top of your dresser.

Sounds
- When interacting with your infant, slow down your speech and over-exaggerate your tone and facial expressions. An infant cannot process auditory information as consistently as an older child, so using fewer

words, spoken at a slower cadence, will allow them to perceive more of what is being said as they are beginning to connect emotion and meaning to the words and tone of voice you use.

- Variety and repetition in auditory stimuli create learning and efficiency in understanding what is being heard. Different environments provide opportunities for varying sounds. To help build your child's awareness, bring their attention to the noises you hear and what those noises mean. For example, your dog's bark will sound different when he is happy and greeting you at the door versus when a stranger is approaching. Point out the sound of a happy bark versus his angry or warning bark.

- Expose your child to a variety of music and instruments. Create the habit of listening to music at certain times during your day or while in the car.

- Expose them to hearing a variety of languages, as well as people of different ages, as the complexity of our speech changes with age and development, so listening to a four-year-old talk versus a forty-year-old is very different.

- Play with different volumes of speech: whisper, shout, sing, talk in funny voices, play with making noises.

- Repeat the noises and babbling and early speech your child makes back to them, mimicking a conversation.

- Talk about what you notice and, when possible, ask questions about what your child hears.

Touch

- Provide exposure to a variety of textures: the feel of a feather when tickling their hands and arms, a soft washcloth, an even softer teddy bear, the smooth surface of a board book. When playing with different toys with your little one, let them experience the different textures on their hands, their cheeks, and even their lips and feet—all places with lots of sensory receptors to process information.

- As your child's language understanding grows, you can begin to share what you notice when holding an object. For example, try saying, "my water bottle is smooth and cold," "the teddy bear is squishy and soft," "the dog is silky and wiggly." Safely explore a range of temperatures: cold, warm, and hot.

- Spend time barefoot on various surfaces, such as the deck, grass, dirt, sand, or the concrete driveway. The bottoms of your feet also have a high concentration of touch receptors, similar to your hands and mouth.

- Get out the play dough, bubbles, sand, water, slime, and food! If there's a food they don't like, let them play with it, even if they won't eat it. Cold cooked broccoli has a smell and texture they can explore, even if they won't put it in their mouth. Play with foods they love, like peanut butter and honey—great things to dig your fingers into then lick them clean (washing them very well both before and after this activity). Take a bowl and fill it with flour, or sugar, or soft butter, and let them feel the differences in the textures and tastes. Tupperware, pots and pans, winter hats and gloves, a pile of books, the laundry basket—all these things may seem boring to us but can create a unique and interesting playtime for kids.

Smells

- Smell everything, everywhere. As you go for a walk, encourage your kids to smell the flowers, the trees, the leaves. As you smell something, talk about it with your kids. If they don't have the ability to answer, share with your kids what you notice. If they can answer, ask them, "What does this smell like to you? What does it remind you of? Do you like the smell?"

- As you're cooking in the kitchen, have your kids smell the various ingredients, herbs, and seasonings. Encourage them to notice how some smells are stronger than others. Ask them if they notice some things that don't have a noticeable smell but still taste delicious.

- Ask, "How about your dog—does he smell fresh and clean, or does he need a bath?" Demonstrating sensory opportunities and engaging in conversation around these experiences will help to create habits as well as increase awareness of these sensory experiences and nuances.

- Don't assume that your child knows how to purposefully smell something. If your child isn't able to comment on smells, holding strong-smelling things close to them for a short while will still expose them to the scent in a way that will contribute to building their ability to perceive different odors over time.

Taste

- Smell and taste work together, and engaging either can enhance both. Even if your infant or child is a picky eater, or particular about taste or texture, you can still encourage them to explore food through sight, touch, and smell, over time working up to taste. You can ease into taste by having your child kiss or lick the food, or telling them they can spit it out after they taste it. You have the rest of their lives to work on table manners, so for now focus on exposure and play to keep mealtimes positive and engaging.

Proprioception (awareness of the body in space) and the vestibular system (which provides information about body movement and rotation)

- Provide opportunities for your infant and toddler to move and be active as often as possible.
- For babies, you can provide the coordinated movements for them while holding their hands or feet. As you're face to face with them, cooing, talking, and entertaining, you can be moving their arms and legs.
- While holding your little one, vary your movements. Jump, hop, dip, twirl, and sway, and they will feel and experience those movements as well.
- As your little one becomes more mobile and stable in their movements, provide varied surfaces for them to sit, crawl, and walk on. The squishiness of a bed, the shifting and uneven surface of sand, the hard surface of the driveway, the itchy feeling of the grass all provide different sensory experiences for the body and movements.
- Run, jump, hop, and walk up hills and down ramps with your child. Have them slide down slides on their bottom, on their tummy, and on their back, each experience a little different from both the sensory and the body awareness perspective (keeping them safe, of course, while doing this).

- Build obstacle courses in your living room or yard requiring your kids to crawl over pillows and under chairs.
- Have your child imitate different animals—cat, dog, elephant, or snake—replicating their movements and noises.
- Play the mirror game, in which your child mirrors your body position or movement. Start with simple examples of movement—stand up, sit down, reach up to the sky—then build in complexity as they are successful mirroring you. Then switch, and you have to imitate or copy your child. Have your child give you feedback as to what you did right or wrong as you mirror their movements.
- Use sidewalk chalk to create lines to walk along or jump over.

Interoception

- Bring awareness to sensations and feelings your child may be experiencing so they can build awareness and understanding. Start simple and basic so they can begin to understand the connections. "You're hot, let's take off your jacket." "Is your tummy telling you that you're hungry and it's time to eat?" "You fell and now you're crying, can you tell me what hurts?"

Elementary School Students

The elementary years can be a time where you hear more about your child's sensory concerns and annoyances. Their increased ability to recognize and verbalize their thoughts and experiences can be both helpful and challenging. Helpful in that they can tell you when they are hungry, rather than bursting into tears, and challenging when they hate what you make for dinner night after night. Continuing to be aware of how sensory experiences impact both your child's day and their overall development can be helpful in learning how to navigate and support this important time of development.

Sensory Development Milestones for Elementary School Students

As the brain continues to develop, kids can more accurately process the more subtle, yet meaningful nuances of sensory experiences. They begin to detect the slight difference in a parent's tone of voice to interpret emotions or to block out background noise in a busy classroom in order to listen and learn. They more quickly process information to follow along more accurately with the teacher talking or the plot in a movie. The continued maturation of the sensory systems supports learning, social interactions, and emotional well-being.

Six to eight years (specific sensory milestones were not found in research or literature for ages nine to twelve):[16]

- Able to handle group situations (e.g., standing in line) without reacting aggressively to being touched
- Has the ability to stay seated (not fidgeting all the time)
- Enjoys playground activities (does not seem fearful when feet leave the ground)
- Comfortable transitioning between activities
- Seems organized in work and play space (not always losing things)
- Able to function in noisy environment

Our elementary-aged kids had several years of sensory exposure and experiences prior to COVID, but they still experienced a sharp reduction of stimuli when the pandemic hit. So, while they'd had more sensory learning under their belt, they still suffered the effects of the void because they were only exposed to the stimuli in their COVID bubble, and they had less layered and varied sensory input. This means that continued and varied sensory exposure is important at all ages, not just in infancy.

To reduce our germ exposure, we cut out the big stuff like going to a major league baseball game, the state fair, concerts, monster truck shows, family trips, and theme parks. There were no adventures away from home with different foods, sights, sounds, and exploration.

We stopped eating out and no longer hosted large parties and gatherings. We didn't make new friends or see people other than close family or neighbors. Entertainment became more technology-based, and we binge-watched shows, hung out on social media, and played video games. We still needed to eat breakfast, lunch, and dinner, but we made these meals at home, went through a drive-thru, or had them delivered rather than eat in crowded restaurants. We all left the house less, which also resulted in wearing pjs and comfy clothes more often and wearing jeans, dresses, and button-down shirts less often.

Upon returning to the classroom, teachers across the country shared differences they saw in kids relative to prior years. Fewer kids were able to tie their shoes. More redirection was needed for more kids to stay on task. More disruptions from upsets and challenging behaviors occurred. The changes in our daily sensory lives contributed to these changes in the kids.

Again, we did what was needed at the time, but applying what we learned will only benefit our kids and families as we work to broaden their horizons and mature their brains.

A great place to start is with food. Eating dinner is a necessity, and if your family eats dinner at home a lot, going out to a restaurant will provide a different sensory experience. Try a new restaurant or visit one you haven't been to in a couple years. The smells, sights, and even the interactions with the servers provide learning experiences for our kids.

I encourage you to eat out as a family, and not just at your local favorite. Be adventurous. Order as a family and try a few new foods in addition to some family favorites. Ask the kids to order for themselves so they can practice speaking up, making eye contact, and interacting with people they don't know. Revel in the music, noise, sights, and smells of the restaurant, then retreat back home to your quiet, familiar space before everyone gets tired and cranky from processing all the stimulation.

Not in the mood to eat out but still interested in providing a sensory experience at dinner? Get creative at home. Change the sensory environment. Eat dinner in the dark with only a few candles lit. Serve pasta, salad, and bread but with no silverware. Provide extra napkins and let the family know that tonight you're eating with your fingers.

Some of my favorite childhood memories are of the nights when we had winter picnics in the living room. We lived in Minnesota, and an indoor picnic on a freezing winter night was a way to change it up for everyone. My dad would build a fire in the fireplace, and my mom would turn down the lights and spread out the picnic on the floor in front of the fire. We'd roast hot dogs and corn on the cob over the fire and make s'mores for dessert. It was simple and inexpensive but created memories that have stayed with me all these years.

Your senses are closely tied to your memories, and when you experience a new, different, or strong sensation—whether it's good or bad—you're more likely to remember the experience. That experience stays with you because it was new and engaged all the senses at the same time. It's a powerful experience for your brain to engage so many regions simultaneously.

The elementary years are a great time to experience bigger events and sensory experiences. Expose kids to those big and layered sensory times and create new memories with big crowds, loud noises, sights, and smells. It doesn't have to be expensive or complicated. Attend a local high school football game or a college lacrosse game. Go watch a 5k or marathon. Get out and do something in a crowd, and experience the noises, smells, and sights you've been missing in the past few years.

If doing new and different things feels overwhelming to you or your kids, it's okay to start small, stay for a short amount of time, and build it up over time. Going to an event for a little while still provides a benefit and sensory exposure. The brain grows and expands when challenged. And you just may be creating that fun family memory your child will carry with them into adulthood.

It's not unusual for a child at this age to be a picky eater—even a *very* picky eater. Interestingly, a study found that sensory sensitivity at age four predicted picky eating at age six.[17] If your child is a picky eater, it may feel like you're on mealtime repeat: cereal for breakfast, mac and cheese for lunch, chicken fingers or cheese pizza for dinner. This is a common repertoire of foods that kids regularly consume. But while it's common, it's far from ideal. Growing brains and bodies require an array of nutrients, and a limited diet doesn't cover all the nutritional bases.

Kids at this age like routine, and they often fight new experiences, which includes eating different foods. It's also a time when they're working to assert their independence, and refusing to eat a food may be one way they use their voices. Don't panic, and know that you're not alone.

In fact, the way Americans ate shifted during the pandemic years—and often not in a good way—and it may have created even more picky eaters.

Because of the increased stress, we relied more heavily on quick and easy processed foods. We were at home all the time as a family, which meant we needed to have much more food on hand. It seemed like the kids didn't stop eating and snacking for most of the day. These quick and easy foods were often packed with flavor, which made a carrot stick or salad even less appealing, and the processed foods were certainly very different in texture than the healthier options.

Picky eating can be tied to development, and you have an opportunity to positively impact your child's eating habits (slowly) by increasing their sensory exposure and development. Providing your child with lots of exposure to smells, tastes, and textures—even if they don't eat the food—can help build familiarity, comfort, and a willingness to eventually eat something new.

One of my favorite stories about picky eating came from a Brain Balance center out west. A family brought their daughter in for help for a variety of reasons: attention, behavior, and picky eating were some of their main concerns—things that impacted the levels of stress and frustration at home. The daughter worked hard through the program, and she had tremendous growth in her development.

At the end of the program, her mom sat down with the Brain Balance director and told example after example of all the positive changes they'd experienced throughout the program. The mom then shared that the one area where she was disappointed was with regard to picky eating; there had been no change.

The director asked the mom what new foods they'd offered the girl, and how it went when they put a new food on the table, or even on her plate.

The mom sat for a moment, then said, "Well, we haven't given her any different foods."

How can you expect your child to try something new if you don't offer it to them?

The mom and the director shared a laugh, then mapped out a plan to try two new foods each week and to document the experience with the daughter using a sticker chart. Now that the daughter had increased maturity in her sensory processing, attention, and behaviors, it was the perfect time to reintroduce foods that hadn't gone well in the past.

The next month the mom was proud to report that the daughter had tried tons of new foods (even more than two each week), and while she didn't like all of them, she had several new foods she was willing, and sometimes even happy, to eat. The lesson here is that kids won't learn and grow without exposure and repetition. And, as parents, we too need to break out of *our* habits to provide different experiences for our kids.

If picky eating is an issue in your household, providing repeated opportunities for smell, taste, and touch will help to mature the awareness, knowledge, and familiarity of the senses involved in eating. It won't happen overnight, but over time, you can expect to see improvement.

Do you remember the first time you ate sushi? For me, the smell of the raw fish combined with the texture was not a hit. But my friends loved it, which meant we went out for sushi often. Each time we went, I'd try a bite. I eventually found the shrimp tempura roll that was crunchy and didn't contain raw fish, then over time I grew to love any and every variety of sushi. It took repeated exposure and experience for me to learn to love something new. It's the same with our kids, but it takes them even more repeated exposure to gain familiarity and comfort in each new experience.

Helping our kids be aware of how they're feeling and be comfortable communicating their thoughts and feelings provides an important tool for life. It's a skill most of us need to continue to develop throughout our lives. Interoception **is your awareness of your internal body and self. It allows you to identify what and how you're feeling and helps you know what to do to support your well-being.** This is considered to be one of the fastest-growing topics in neuroscience and psychology today. Professor Manos Tsakiris, a psychologist at Royal Holloway, University of London, states, "We are seeing an exponential growth in interoception research." One finding is that "Scientists have shown that our sensitivity to interoceptive signals can determine our capacity to regulate our emotions, and our subsequent susceptibility to mental health problems such as anxiety and depression."[18] The more aware we are of our sensations and feelings, the better we tend to do in reacting to and handling those feelings.

When I'm irritable, I try to first notice that I'm cranky, then stop and evaluate the situation. Am I well rested and well fed? If I'm tired or hungry,

I'm much more likely to be irritable and to react in an exaggerated manner. If I take note of how I feel, it gives me information about what I can do to feel better. When I'm tired and irritable, eating, sleeping, or exercising can turn my mood around. If I'm feeling stressed or overwhelmed with how much I need to accomplish in a day, creating a to-do list and a plan can help me feel more in control. It's up to parents to foster this awareness and knowledge—this interoception—in our kids.

We had a growth moment of interoception with our son, Drew, during the pandemic.

He was in fourth grade when school closed a week early for spring break, and then the closure was extended significantly while the school worked to put a distance learning plan in place. School did eventually continue, but as partial days of virtual learning. Then it was summer break.

This was the largest chunk of unstructured time that my kids had ever had. They were part of a year-round school system, and prior to this, the longest break they'd ever had was for five weeks over the summer. They played multiple sports and were involved in various activities. And I'm a social person, so I loved to make plans with friends and family. Like most other families, we were on the go constantly. Having almost five months without structure was alarming, and we weren't prepared to fill that void of time.

At the same time, work for both Doug and me went into overdrive. The result was bored kids and preoccupied parents. Our daughter, an avid reader, read more books than ever, and our son suddenly had access to gaming in a way we'd never previously allowed.

You can probably guess where this was heading.

I *knew* that hours of video games was not good for his mood, behavior, or development. But I also knew we were in a unique time that we just needed to get through. I also naively thought it would be over soon.

Most of the time, Drew was a chill, happy kid. He'd always done an amazing job entertaining himself. He'd wander outside; find a friend; grab a hockey stick, racket, ball, bike, fishing pole, dog, or anything else; and play. Then he'd wander back inside, grab some food, tell me a story, and head back out to do it again.

But now he couldn't play with the neighbors, and he began saying, "I'm bored. This sucks." Over and over. We didn't disagree. Nor were we surprised to hear he was bored. We all were.

Drew was playing Fortnite without supervision, and there were prearranged times when he'd connect with his cousin, Ollie, in Minnesota, so they could play together. We thought it was great that he and Ollie, whom he considers one of his best friends, were connecting each day.

He also had days and times he would connect with friends from school to play.

We began to notice that Drew was turning negative—extremely negative. He snapped back at us and complained about everything. We were slow on the uptake. The gaming continued, and so did his sour mood.

When we started noticing even more intense behaviors, meltdowns, and anxiety, we intervened. Drew hadn't displayed anxious behaviors in the past, and while we could understand having fears and anxiety around the pandemic, it still felt out of character. So we sat down with him and talked about how his behavior seemed to correlate with his increase in gaming.

Of course, he fought back on this idea. We agreed to try a week without playing video games at all, just to see if it made a difference. While he pouted and had an attitude the first day or two, by the end of the week, Drew seemed more himself.

We sat down again to talk about how he was now feeling and behaving, and the conversation was telling. Drew said that when he took a break from the game, he realized that playing it made him feel "really intense." He was super focused and competitive, so trying to earn points, to get the other players eliminated, and to go for the Victory Royale—the big win in the game—made him tense. Even when he was finished playing for the day, he kept feeling really intense. He said he didn't like that feeling, and that since he'd stopped playing, he felt a *little* better.

Drew still wanted to be able to play with Ollie and his friends, so we agreed to revert back to our pre-pandemic rules: no gaming during the week, and an hour each day on the weekend. Tops.

This schedule worked well for the next few months, and eventually Drew just stopped playing. The parent in me would like to think it was because he felt better not playing, but the truth is he probably got bored with the game. Either way, it felt like a big win. Drew recognized how he was feeling, was able to talk about it, and then was willing to make a change to support his well-being. I thought that was pretty impressive for a fourth grader.

Sensory Development Activities for Elementary School Students

Even if your child is elementary age, be sure to review the activity suggestions for infants and toddlers as well.

Ways to engage each sense
Remember, it doesn't need to be fancy or elaborate for it to be a new and beneficial sensory experience. Elementary-aged kids can tolerate sensory stimulation for longer periods of time with more layered experiences. This is a great age for family adventures that provide both new and favorite experiences and activities for your kids. Continue to focus on both variety and repetition to contribute to your child's sensory learning experience and development.

Sight
- Be sure to get your kids out of the house. Have them spend time with groups of kids in the neighborhood, the park, place of worship, community center, or skate park.
- Have your child engage in physical activities like sports as well as enriching activities like acting, cooking, or art.
- Visit parks, trails, libraries, museums, and stores.
- Bring your kids to an outdoor store that sells camping and fishing gear and be patient to allow them time to spend exploring the store and gear. Then have your kids help plan an adventure where they can use the gear or equipment. Plan a camping night in the backyard or a fishing outing at a local pond.
- Encourage your kids to think about a variety of nature sights they could experience: streams, ponds, lakes, oceans, fields, hills, mountains. Create lists of things they have and have not experienced,

then work to check those items off the list! See a falling star at night, catch a firefly in early summer, pick dandelions in the yard, smell the leaves on a trail in the fall. Each one of those experiences provides differing sensory input.

Sounds

- Nature, kids, adults, animals: each creates different noises for the brain to process and identify. Attend events with big crowds like the state fair, an outdoor concert, sporting events, or parades. Experiment with a variety of different types of music and instruments. Establish a habit of listening to music at certain times during your day or while in the car.

- Listen to podcasts and audiobooks in the car. The books you remember enjoying as a child can be re-experienced together while running errands.

- Play games where you listen to a commercial and need to count the number of times you hear a certain word, try to repeat the commercial, or make up your own version of how you would sell that product.

Touch

- Arts, crafts, building, and cooking are great ways to experience a variety of touch sensations while working on coordination, focus, and planning skills.

- Encourage your kids to get outside and catch frogs, dig for worms, then go fishing.

- Allow them to get their hands dirty by planting and caring for a garden.

- Have your kids spend time barefoot on various surfaces, even as the kids get older—the deck, grass, dirt, sand, the concrete driveway. Make your own play dough, bubbles, slime, or snacks. Have an occasional meal without silverware or establish times where it's okay for your kids to play with their food.

Smells

- Smell everything, everywhere! Talk to your kids about what they smell: Do they like it? Does it remind them of anything or trigger a particular memory or feeling?

- Incorporate smell into as many activities as you can—if your child is taking a bath, add a few drops of an essential oil or diffuse an oil during homework time. While you're cooking, have your child smell the various ingredients, then notice if it smells the same or different when combined with other ingredients, and then baked.

Taste

- Remember that taste and smell work together, and engaging either can enhance both.
- This is a great age to broaden their horizons with introducing new foods. Each time you're at a restaurant, have them try a bite of what you have ordered. Talk about the food first: Do they like the smell? Do they think it will taste like it smells? How do they like the look of it? Is it boring, or pretty, or does it remind them of something else they've eaten? Make a game of it—do they like it the same, better, or worse than what they ordered?
- Many kids are picky eaters at this age, but you can help them build comfort and familiarity with different foods through repeated exposures and getting them used to the sights, smells, and textures of new things. If they won't eat a food, throw out the rules and have them play with it and smell it. Or try just one bite each time; even if they spit it out, they are tasting and chewing it, building up that repeated exposure.
- Work together with your child to create a list of new and different foods to try. You can take a stroll through your neighborhood grocery store or an ethnic store you haven't visited before to help provide ideas of things to try.
- Have your child page through a cookbook or website that provides both recipes and lists of ingredients. Then, after trying the new foods, create a list of things they loved and hated. Both experiences are good, as they are still providing sensory adventures.

Proprioception (awareness of the body in space) and the vestibular system (which provides information about body movement and rotation)

- Encourage your kids to be physically active with varied activities. Riding a bike creates different sensations of balance and movement and requires different types of body coordination than riding a scooter.

- Going for a long walk requires different movements than playing freeze tag, which requires sprinting and then holding completely still.
- Swinging on a swing and swaying back and forth in a hammock are also similar yet different movements and sensations.
- Kids love to do what they are good at, but growth happens when something is a little challenging. If they're good a rollerblading, try ice skating. If they're good at soccer, try playing ultimate frisbee. If their balance is good, try paddling on a stand-up paddle board. Be creative and adventurous.
- Play games that require specific body movements, such as hopscotch, Simon says, Twister, cat's cradle (using string), and charades.
- Spinning a hula hoop, jumping on a pogo stick, and dribbling a basketball all also require awareness and control of body movements to be successful.
- Jump rope and, as they improve, watch YouTube videos of the amazing tricks kids can do with jump ropes.
- Watch a TikTok dance video together, then make one together.
- Walk on a curb or balance beam, and once they have mastered it, try new movements that continue to challenge their balance.
- Record a video of your child the first time they try a new physical activity, then again a few weeks later so they can watch the difference and improvements that happen over time!
- Keep in mind what we learned about the RAS—the first time your child tries something new, it will be more stressful and will drain more resources, but over time and with repetition the brain will learn and become more automated, calm, and efficient in the experience. So, just because your child doesn't like doing something new on the first try doesn't mean you should give it up.

Interoception
- Bringing awareness to sensations and feelings your kids may be experiencing, on a level they can understand, can help to build their awareness as well. You can kindly point out what you are observing

in them: "I'm noticing that you are really tired right now, so the loud noises your brother is making are irritating you"; or "You seem stressed. Are you worried about your math homework? Let's do it together so we can get it out of the way, then play a game when we're done."

- You can also model by sharing what you are experiencing: "I'm having a hard time deciding what I want to eat right now because I waited too long and am so hungry I can't think"; or "I'm feeling crabby right now because I am stressed with the amount of work I have to do tonight."

Create family adventures

- Go to ethnic restaurants, anything different from your daily norm: Vietnamese, Thai, Italian, Ethiopian, Irish, Mexican, Japanese.
- Choose a new favorite ethnic cuisine or dish and try to make it at home.
- Have a taste test contest at home where you all taste several different things and rate them on smell, taste, and presentation.
- Visit different religious services and notice the differences in the music, the routines of the service, the look of the building.
- Create new experiences: try fishing, skiing, canoeing, rock climbing, running a race, or watching a marathon. When you do something new, talk about your sensory experience: What did you hear, see, smell, experience? How does it make you feel? (For example, watching a marathon is so inspiring but also hard. You see the pain and agony but also the joy when the runner crosses the finish line. Does that inspire you to want to run a marathon?)

Middle School and High School Students

With development comes an increase in endurance. For sensory experiences, this means an ability to process larger amounts of information for longer periods of time before the resources needed to process this information are depleted, resulting in frustration, irritation, or shutdown. This can look like the ability to enjoy a loud and chaotic event, such as a professional sporting event, for a longer period of time. Or the ability to block out sensory distractions for a sustained period of time to remain focused on homework to study for a test or write a paper. Immaturities in sensory processing for these ages can present as a shorter fuse for handling frustrations and less of an ability to sustain focus on necessary tasks.

Sensory Development Milestones for
Middle School and High School Students

While there aren't specific sensory milestones for kids at this age, the expectation is that kids are able to tolerate and process more sensory input for longer periods of time, and that their awareness of how they feel has increased. **This increased awareness allows kids to begin to make intentional choices for self-regulation, such as choosing to spend time on their own if feeling irritable or overwhelmed or asking you to turn down the music in the car if it is too much for them in that moment.**

The pandemic impacted every age group in different ways. Cutting off social interactions for our teens meant interrupting a defining cornerstone of this age—socialization with peers. As teens strive toward independence and finding their place in the world, they naturally venture farther away from their home base and form deep and meaningful connections with peers and romantic interests. Closed off in bedrooms across the country, teens engaged significantly more in screen time during the pandemic—a combination of virtual school, TikTok, YouTube, Snapchat, video gaming, FaceTime, and more. For teens, technology became the thread and connection to peers, with a reported 50% to 70% increase in technology usage.[19] That increase translates to approximately five hours *more* screen time *per day* than before the pandemic.[20] For "heavy users," that totals 17.5 hours of screen time per day. You read that correctly. That barely leaves time for anything else— adequate sleep, meals, or movement. Of the increase in screen time, 50% of the tech time was on social media. While those numbers dropped somewhat once kids were back in school, they remain alarmingly higher than they were pre-pandemic.

In the wake of pandemic changes and technology usage, there have been some horrifying statistics about soaring rates of ADHD, anxiety, depression, and teen suicide. The CDC's "Morbidity and Mortality Weekly Report" stated a 22.3% increase in emergency room trips for potential suicides in ages twelve to seventeen in 2020 compared to 2019.[21] While researchers caution against blaming the pandemic for the sharp increase (and technology alone is not to blame), it's a piece of the puzzle in understanding and supporting the well-being of teenagers.

Using technology engages some senses, sight and sound, but not as many of the senses as other experiences. Critical elements left out are body movements (providing proprioception), smell, light touch beyond the hands, and interoception—your awareness of your body, your movements, and how you are feeling.

While it is easy to lump all types of technology into one category, there are differences between scrolling through social media on your phone and gaming. In addition to the lack of movement involved in gaming, a large amount of fuel is burned to support the visual processing load of a video game and the intense, sustained engagement. And as the brain is depleted of fuel, it naturally shifts to more negative moods and emotions. Further, when kids are fatigued, there can be an increase in impulsive behaviors and less control, focus, and regulation.

To help counter the increase in tech usage, we need to create a structure to help our teens balance technology with physical activity and face-to-face interactions with peers. While this is easier said than done, keeping your child involved in activities can be helpful. Busy kids have less downtime to spend on technology and will have more time to spend with friends, engaging their senses.

One of my friends reached out to me during the pandemic. Her brilliant son Jack was struggling. With changes in school and life, he spent all his time in the basement gaming. He was moody and irritable, picked fights at home, and was failing his classes. My friend was concerned and rightfully so. While she knew that gaming and time spent on YouTube weren't productive, when she tried to control how he spent his time, it resulted in fights that could be explosive and were upsetting and disruptive to the whole family.

I spent some time with Jack and quickly realized it wasn't only his mom who was upset. He was miserable. He didn't feel good about failing classes, but he didn't have the energy or desire to do anything different. He said, "I have no life. What else am I supposed to do all day, or when I can't sleep at night?"

Jack agreed to do the Brain Balance home program with me to see if it could help get him back on track with school and maybe even feeling a little better. While this program is normally done with a live coach on the computer, because I lived nearby, we did it in person, meeting a few times a week in our open garage. It got Jack up and out of the house in the morning and moving three times a week. During the program, he received lots of sensory stimulation while doing core and eye exercises and working on his balance. I did the exercises with Jack and have to admit that I not only enjoyed it but I benefited greatly in my mood and productivity too.

Beyond the program days, Jack and I mapped out a plan for him to get outside to exercise several days a week. It didn't need to be anything too crazy. Just a 20-minute bike ride would be great. Jack committed to our plan and was consistent with meeting me to do the program and with exercising some on his own.

At the end of his program, Jack gave me one of the best compliments. He told me he didn't want to be finished and wished he could keep going. The combination of connecting while doing the exercises (we truly had so much fun: good music, exercise, and laughter were so beneficial to both of us during that lockdown period), paired with the brain, body, and visual exercises and sensory stimulation, made a difference for Jack. He could feel the difference and didn't want it to end.

He got his grades back on track and was getting along better at home. We talked through his plans going forward to continue on this positive path, and I reminded him about the importance of staying active, engaging the senses, connecting with friends, and not gaming for hours on end. Several months later I was thrilled to hear that, on his own, Jack found a yoga group to join with his peers and he started attending weekly.

While doing the program together, Jack and I spent a lot of time talking about what we were doing and why. Why exercise is important to the brain and body, and the signs and clues your brain gives you so you can make choices to support feeling and functioning at your best.

Interoception, awareness of yourself, is not easy at any age, but hopefully

Jack's experience at this young age is one he'll continue to learn and grow from. The ability to identify how you are feeling and why, then what you can do to shift how you are feeling, is a lifelong tool for success and wellness, and one that doesn't develop easily.

Beyond balancing technology with movement and interactions to help support your teens, providing face-to-face interactions and connections with friends and family is so important to foster a sense of community and well-being.[22] Find an activity outside of school to help your child engage with their peers. Sports, a religious youth group, a yoga class, a cooking class, theater, art, volunteering—anything. When a child is actively engaged in an activity, they're out of their room, moving around, and having more opportunity to form the connections they crave. If the first few groups or activities you try aren't the right fit, don't give up. Connect with the school counselor for recommendations on clubs, activities, or even other kids who may be good friends to get to know.

I'll never forget a conversation I had several years ago with an administrator at a Florida university. He talked about the importance of getting incoming freshmen involved in activities within the first 30 days at school. He stressed that getting kids connected and engaged significantly reduces dropout rates and supports mental well-being during a major transition period. People are happier and healthier when they are connected and involved.

Beyond building connections and relationships, keeping your child physically active can have a grounding, soothing effect through engaging proprioception, in addition to the other benefits of cardio exercise on mood and mental state. Joints and muscles in your body have receptors that are activated through movement. When there's movement or pressure, the receptor sends a message to the brain relaying that information. Stimulation to the brain wakes it up. Activities like running, jumping, balancing, and moving provide stimulation to these receptors. Proprioception is what allows you to close your eyes and still touch your finger to your nose, even though you can't see your nose or your finger. You simply know because of this sense.

We are vaguely aware of our body at all times. Close your eyes, and you can still describe the position you're sitting in, how your legs are crossed, and the way your hands are holding the tablet or book. Now pay attention to what you are *most* aware of. For me, I'm most aware of where my left leg is crossed over my right knee and where my bum and low back are against the chair. Wherever there's pressure, I'm more aware of those areas because of proprioception.

To try this, sit with your eyes closed and your feet flat on the ground. Then cross one leg over the other and notice your heightened awareness. Now, shake your foot and notice how movement *increases* your awareness of your foot. That is proprioception in action.

Not everyone is equal in their proprioceptive awareness. An injury, like a sprained ankle, can be disruptive to proprioception in a joint. There are also times when aspects of development are immature, resulting in a reduction in awareness. Kids and adults who struggle with proprioception may tend to appear more clumsy. They can also experience heightened levels of stress and anxiety, feelings of disconnection from their body, and social challenges. Our social interactions are highly dependent on our ability to pick up on social cues and clues through body language and facial expressions. To understand body language in someone else, you first need to be able to identify it in yourself, and if you aren't able to sense your body, you aren't aware of your facial expression and posture when you're angry versus confused. The differences are small but important. Your ability to see and understand social cues and interactions is in part dependent on accurate proprioception.

One example of proprioception in action is the use of weighted blankets. These special blankets increase external pressure on the body, heightening your awareness of your body, which can be soothing and comforting. Kids who are immature in aspects of development often struggle with proprioception and have less awareness of their body and movements. The weight of the blanket provides stronger input to the brain than a traditional blanket. While this can be a comforting strategy to employ, it may be a red flag that the sensory processing for this child is disrupted, requiring stronger input to process.

Any movement that uses your joints—or applies pressure to your joints and muscles—activates this sensory information system in your body. Go for a jog, grab a jump rope, bounce on a trampoline. It doesn't need to be fancy or prolonged. While there are benefits to extended exercise, proprioception input doesn't require long stretches of time. In fact, short intervals throughout the day can be effective in providing this grounding sensory input.

I know firsthand how hard it can be to drag a teenager out of bed to come downstairs and engage with the family, let alone exercise.

We were so thrilled when our school decided to continue cross-country in the fall of the 2021–22 school year. Morgan had been part of the team the year before, and while it's a brutal sport of pushing through pain and discomfort, it's a team-training environment and exercise. Outside. With friends.

I know the difference a run can have on my own mood and energy, and it never ceases to amaze me how it impacts the kids (remember the water-skiing example with Ely?). You'd think that after a long day of school, running several miles in the North Carolina heat would exhaust the kids. Day after day, they'd get in the car after practice and be chattier and more engaged than when I picked them up right after school. Cross-country practice was like a jolt of caffeine. By the end of the night, they were tired and sore, and they would sleep in as long as humanly possible on the weekends, but after practice, they were happy and engaged.

Sensory Development Activities for Middle School and High School Students

Don't forget to review previous examples shared for infants and toddlers and elementary-aged kids.

Ways to engage each sense

At this age, focus on finding ways to create sensory-rich activities while creating new experiences, strengthening connections with friends, and working to incorporate more movement and exercise to help balance technology time.

To help immerse middle school and older kids in an experience, I encourage you to do something that may feel counterintuitive. I *want* the kids to take out their phones and take pictures! The key is to not snap aimlessly, but to engage at a deeper level in the moment. The book *Peak Mind* by Dr. Amishi Jha shares research to answer the question: Can you be truly present in a moment when you're snapping photos? The answer is more complex than a simple *yes* or *no*. People who snap pictures are less likely to remember the moment than those who aren't taking photos. However, you could *increase* your likelihood of recalling the moment by taking a photo and focusing on a particular detail in that photo.[23] So, the key to remembering something is to either experience the moment without taking pictures—to be present and soak up the sensory details—or to take pictures as long as you're tuned in to a specific detail. So let your kids snap away and encourage them to capture something special or unique in each photo.

Layered sensory experiences
- Help your teen create a de-stressing routine that includes all the senses: light a favorite candle, turn down the lights, turn on nature sounds or something soothing, add a cozy blanket, and practice meditation with a meditation app.
- Other ways to experience layered sensory experiences at this age include attending a high school football game and encouraging your student to notice all the elements: the dark fall night, the cool and crisp air, the sound of the crowd cheering and football pads smacking together, the taste of popcorn and soda.
- Find new and different experiences you can do as a family or they could do with a friend, like running a 5k or entering a triathlon, hiking a mountain, or having a scavenger hunt through downtown.

Sight
- Get your teenager out of the house to explore. Have them create or find a list of the top hikes in your area, then explore and rate which hikes have the best views.
- Visit a variety of ethnic grocery stores and explore the different produce and food options.
- Find a local farmer's market and notice the differences in what is offered seasonally.

- Visit coffee shops throughout town and rate them based on ambiance, decor, and which has the best games available (or any games available).
- During the holidays, download a scavenger hunt list to explore the holiday lights in your area.
- If your teen rejects all your ideas, have them come up with their own list of experiences and adventures.

Sounds

- Explore different genres of music.
- Play an instrument; whether they play poorly or exceptionally well, it still provides auditory stimulation.
- Find a podcast you can listen to together in the car that sparks a conversation or debate you can engage in together after listening.
- Listen to an audiobook, or several, in the car and note the differences in the narrators and background music and how they add to the listening experience.
- Talk about how different times of day or times of year can sound different.
- The stillness outside after a fresh snow in the winter, the rustling of the leaves in the wind in the spring, the crunching of brittle leaves in the fall, or the cicadas singing in the heat and humidity of summer: even if your teen is ignoring you, pointing out these sensory experiences still may heighten their awareness and appreciation.
- Listen to the varying tones and rhythms of different languages.
- Talk about their sport or hobby and the auditory cues they use in their sport—while running, can they hear a runner approaching them from behind? Do they listen to their coach shouting from the sidelines of a soccer game while blocking out the directions from the parents also shouting from the sidelines?
- Talk about which noises are peaceful and relaxing versus which noises are stressful.
- Discuss how music in the background while studying at this age can be helpful or disruptive depending on their level of focus in that

moment, and when and how they can use or avoid music to help them study.

Touch

- I love encouraging kids this age to spend time in the kitchen. Have your kids cook, chop, dice, mix, and make sushi rolls. For a baking project, have them crack and separate eggs, knead dough, cut out and frost cookies, decorate a cake, or make homemade cannoli.
- If cooking isn't something you can talk them into doing, try crafts: painting, drawing, chalk art, pottery, clay, knitting, sanding and repainting a piece of furniture, learning to sew.
- Have them build something: a birdhouse, a shelf, an obstacle course in the backyard for yourself, or even a squirrel obstacle course (search YouTube for ideas—it's really a thing!).
- They could plant an herb garden.
- Experiment with makeup and painting finger and toenail designs.
- Learn how to throw a frisbee or a boomerang, or play jacks, dominoes, or Jenga.

Smells

- Create a routine for homework time for your student that involves using a favorite essential oil. As you cook in the kitchen, have your child smell the various ingredients, herbs, and seasonings. Have your teen create homemade drinks and smoothies that incorporate both smell and taste (for example, strawberry mint water).

Taste

- Visit ethnic restaurants as a family.
- Have your kids try the same flavor of ice cream at several different ice cream shops to compare the differences.
- Visit several different coffee shops over time, ordering the same drink and comparing how a chai tea at Starbucks tastes completely different than one from Caribou Coffee, then rate your favorites and try to re-create them at home for a fraction of the price.
- Create a blind taste test at home where family members try to identify different bubbly waters or sodas by taste.
- Have a family cook-off and see who makes the best muffins.

Proprioception (awareness of the body in space)

- Encourage your kids to move. Remember that input into the joints and muscles provides input into the brain, which can be both energizing and comforting to the brain.
- Have your kids stay involved in team sports, and if team sports isn't the thing for your child, keep working to find something that is— yoga, Pilates, rock climbing, skateboarding, trampolining, mountain biking, golf, pickleball, kayaking, canoeing, swimming. Anything that involves the muscles and movement can be beneficial.
- At this age kids are often much more willing to do something active if they can do it with a friend. Have your kids create a list with their friends of physical activities in your area they'd be willing to do.

Interoception

Interoception may be one of the hardest senses to develop awareness around but one of the most powerful tools to have in life—an awareness of what you are feeling and why. There is so much you can't control in life, but there are some things you can control that can have a direct impact on how you feel.

- To continue to help your teenagers build awareness of themselves and how they feel, encourage practice of a progressive relaxation or mindfulness meditation. These are powerful strategies to build awareness. Help your teen find and work into their daily routine the use of a meditation app and/or a guided progressive relaxation.
- Encourage your child to practice deep belly breathing, concentrating on breathing into the stomach instead of the chest to help restore calm and relaxation in moments of stress.
- Continue to model what you notice within yourself and the action step you're taking because of what you noticed. "I'm starting to get a headache, which made me realize I haven't eaten since breakfast, so I'm going to grab a protein snack." "I'm in such a negative mood today, but I didn't sleep well last night, so I know being tired is making my mood worse, I'm going to go for a walk to help energize my mood and brain."
- Gently point out in your kids what you are noticing and offer to support them in that moment. "I'm sensing you're feeling edgy right

now. Are you feeling overwhelmed with your workload tonight? How can I help?"

Signs That Indicate Improvement

When there's a change to how your child's brain is processing sensory information, so many things can be impacted. These changes can be subtle and easy to miss, as it is often easier to notice the start of something new rather than something slowly fading away. Changes often begin with increased tolerance. In a toddler, you may notice they begin tolerating clothing better, and they keep their socks, shoes, or any article of clothing on longer than before. You may notice less complaining and irritation with tags and textures of clothing. Your child may start commenting on smells or become a little less dramatic with the smells they don't like. They may begin to tolerate being in a noisy, crowded place for longer before reaching their limit and getting crabby. Your child may start to become less reactive to loud noises such as fireworks or the vacuum cleaner or hand dryers in public restrooms. As their sensory perception continues to improve, you'll eventually notice an increased willingness to try new and different foods—and they may even like them. In teenagers you may notice them beginning to self-regulate, to make choices to take a break from a chaotic sensory experience, or to do physical activity as a way to feel better.

Some of the most subtle yet most important changes will impact mood and anxiety. Remember, our senses orient us in the world. They allow us to process what's happening all around us and how it impacts us. "I hear a noise. Is something coming toward me? I see a ball someone threw my way. Should I duck or try to catch it?" When your senses are dialed in, you can more accurately understand what's happening in the world around you and prepare to act or react as needed. Maturity in the sensory system can contribute to a calmer, more relaxed, and more tolerant mood and an expanded capacity to handle a more chaotic environment with ease.

3
....

FINE MOTOR DEVELOPMENT

Have you ever experienced whining, avoidance, or a flare-up in frustrating behaviors when it was time to get out the pencil and paper? Or do your kids avoid wearing certain clothing—items that require buttons, zippers, or laces? Does your high school student hate writing papers and do anything they can to avoid it? These behaviors can be red flags that your child may be struggling with fine motor skills. When fine motor skills are immature, children need to work *harder* and put in more effort to accomplish what seem like simple tasks. And that's not fun.

Fine motor skills **translates to small muscle movements—which apply not only to the hands but to other critical areas as well. Both speech and coordinated eye movements also require intricate coordination of many small muscles and timing to be successful.** Remember the marionette? Like the puppeteer, the brain is orchestrating these delicate movements.

Behaviors such as avoidance tactics and even melting down can flare up when handwriting is hard, and you can see challenges and resistance when speech and eye movements are difficult too. When speech is hard, communicating when frustrated or upset becomes even more difficult, which can result in tears. Immaturity in eye coordination can interfere with reading, comprehension, and other work in the classroom, resulting in a dislike of reading or school.

Disruptions in neural development involving fine motor coordination can result in complications that impact learning and social interactions. When a task is difficult, extra effort and energy are required to attempt the task, which can leave kids drained and frustrated, but increasing fine motor skills can help reduce the frustrations.

Note to Parents

Some of your child's frustrating behaviors could be masking underlying challenges with fine motor skills. All of us become more negative and irritable when asked to do a task we don't feel we have the resources to do. This may be happening for your child, resulting in feelings of being overwhelmed or incapable.

Clues that indicate immature fine motor skills for the hands include: grasping the pencil firmly to maintain control, pushing harder than necessary when writing, making large or irregular letters, using inconsistent spacing, or taking a long time to complete the task.

Difficulties with speech can present as delays in beginning to babble and speak, issues with enunciation, struggles to be understood by people outside the immediate family, or a tendency to answer questions with a minimal response.

Immature coordination of eye movements can present as missed problems on a worksheet, a dislike of reading, or a hard time taking notes in class. Disruptions in smooth, controlled eye movements can be harder for parents to detect than speech difficulties or an altered pencil grasp.

Working to enhance your child's fine motor skills—for the hands, mouth, and eyes—even if they're older, can help improve task efficiency and minimize the effort and frustration that may accompany those tasks—allowing them to redirect resources toward attention, managing behaviors, and learning.

While there's a big emphasis on fine motor skills for hands and speech in preschool and early elementary years, the need for those skills doesn't go away when the child gets older, although there's less opportunity to practice and less support to develop the skills. And while eye movements happen constantly throughout the day, that doesn't mean they are accurate or efficient. This means, even if your child is older, you should still pay attention to these three categories of fine motor skills.

As parents, we have so many reasons to worry about our kids, and their fine motor skills don't often make the top of the list. While a person can live a happy and fulfilled life without stellar handwriting, ease and accuracy of speech and sustained eye movements make a huge difference in daily life. By working to support your child's foundational development, you will in turn help to maximize development in these more complex and involved tasks, which will deliver improved outcomes with less effort.

Pandemic Lessons

Increased usage of technology at young ages has had an impact on the emerging fine motor skills of our infants and toddlers, resulting in less time coloring and drawing and more time staring at a device held in their hands.[1] While technology requires some hand fine motor movements—children must swipe a tablet screen or tap an object to select it—and eye movements, swiping a screen does *not* require the same level of coordination and nuance that will eventually be needed to take notes in class and hold a pencil.

Preliminary research in 2022 from Gerry Giesbrecht, PhD, a psychologist with the Department of Pediatrics at the University of Calgary, found that infants born during the pandemic had nearly twice the likelihood of experiencing developmental delays in social and communication development.[2] Students at Brain Balance were testing up to 15% lower than pre-pandemic times in fine motor skills. They also had lower scores in tasks requiring auditory, visual, and motor responses.

The activities and stimulation for kids during the pandemic shifted, which impacted their development. But knowledge is power, and knowing the hurdles in front of us gives us an opportunity to address them. Neuroplasticity means the brain can change, and with a plan in place, you can support your child's development to get them back on track and minimize their frustrations—and yours too. Begin by addressing the underlying function, the fine motor skills, then use play to practice. It can be a fun and effective way to drive improvement for your child.

All fine motor skills begin with simple coordination and layer in complexity and control over time. An infant grasps your extended finger or a toy, a one-year-old will work on the pincer grasp to pick up a Cheerio or bite of food, a toddler will grab a crayon to color, a six-year-old will learn to tie their shoes, and older students write words, sentences, and eventually papers. Fine motor skills, like other aspects of development, require the integration of many separate functions that layer together to develop a more complex skill or ability. Over time, this results in skill and control.

The foundation of fine motor skills begins with the development of gross motor functions—large muscles build strength and coordination—then progresses to the smaller muscles that are involved in small, sequenced movements. If a child is behind in developing their large motor muscle groups, it can delay the layered development of the fine motor muscles and coordination.

With speech, an infant starts with sucking and swallowing, then progresses to finding their voice through play with noise and babbling. Eventually consonant sounds emerge, "dadada," and over time, with increased fine-tuned control, those babbles become words and then sentences (there is so much more to developing speech than this short paragraph, but the goal is to illustrate that development moves from simple to complex over time).

An infant's eyes start by seeing stark contrast with black and white and then begin to be able to focus on an object at close range, such as a parent's face.[3] Over the next few months babies begin to develop a bit more control and start to shift their eyes between two things or to follow a moving object with their eyes. With time, practice, and efficiency the eyes can scan across a line of text to read quickly or shift from near to far—then return to the precise place the eyes left off, for example, to quickly take notes in class.

The progression of fine motor development for the hands happens through stimulation of touch, exposure to new and different tasks, then practice and repetition. Much of the exposure and practice happens naturally for children. They seek out a ball and practice picking it up and dropping it, which teaches them how much pressure they need to exert to hold the ball and how to change their grip to drop it. Learning the pincer grasp happens when a baby wants to pick something up and put it in their mouth to either eat or explore the object. Their drive and curiosity are naturally there if given the right direction and opportunity.

Beyond natural drive and curiosity, early school also provides a great deal of structured teaching and practice for development. Tracing shapes, cutting with scissors, looking at a letter, tracking across letters to read a word, and learning to pronounce letter sounds and count syllables are all ways that fine motor skills for hands, speech, and eyes are practiced in school.

Later school years build on these foundations as students write essays instead of letters, read paragraphs and chapters rather than just words, and communicate thoughts and ideas in a concise manner through speech and writing. Complications in foundational skills will interfere with success in the abilities expected of older students.

If your child is presenting with frustrations or deficits in any of these areas, going back to the basics and building from there will help to ease the challenge.

Science Alert

Fine motor skills require many small muscles to work together with perfect coordination and timing. The improvement in the synchronization of these motor skills happens through two important processes in the brain, allowing actions to be faster and more complex. These advances happen through *myelination* and *pruning*. Myelination is the insulation, or covering, that forms around neuron axons to support fast communication between the nerves, and pruning is the natural process that eliminates extra connections in the brain. The textbook *Peripheral Neuropathy* has a chapter dedicated to myelination; it states, "Pruning is our body's way of maintaining more efficient brain functions as we get older and learn new complex information."[4] The infant brain experiences an explosion in growth, building new connections. Then, by ages two to three, the brain begins to selectively eliminate connections that aren't needed.

Picture driving from your house to a location across town. There are several different routes you could take to get there, but taking the highway, rather than the dirt road that is out of the way, is the most efficient plan. Pruning is the brain's way of removing the dirt roads as options, leaving only the fastest and best routes.

Stimulation and repetition guide pruning in the brain. Less variety of experiences, or less repetition, will lead to less pruning, and a brain that is less efficient in coordinating networks of nerves to work together.

> Think of everything that's involved in tying your shoes. You have to both remember and execute a series of complex events: crossing one lace over another, wrapping it around, tucking it back through, then pulling tight while holding on to the other lace so it doesn't pull through. There's a lot that goes into tightly tied shoes. Over time, through repetition and practice, this complex task becomes automated, requiring minimal effort thanks to myelination and pruning.

Infants and Toddlers

Fine motor skills don't start with the ability to pick up a Cheerio or write your name. They begin with body awareness, sensory stimulation, and movement, then refine over time through use and practice. Understanding how this progression works can help you stimulate and guide healthy development to keep things on track from the start.

Fine Motor Development Milestones for Infants and Toddlers

Hands[5]

Four months:
- Brings hands to mouth

Nine months:
- Moves things from one hand to another
- Bangs two objects together
- Uses fingers to "rake" food toward self

Twelve months:
- Picks up things such as Cheerios with thumb and pointer finger
- Can put an object in a container

Fifteen months:
- Begins to stack two objects
- Tries to use objects, like a phone, cup, or book, correctly

Eighteen months:
- Feeds self with fingers
- Tries to use a spoon
- Scribbles with a crayon

Two years:
- Plays with buttons
- Switches knobs on a toy (turning it off/on)
- Holds an object in one hand while using the other hand, like when taking a lid off a cup
- Eats with a spoon

Thirty months:
- Uses hands to twist doorknobs, unscrew a lid
- Can turn pages in a book one at a time
- Can take some clothes off independently, such as pants or a jacket

Three years:
- Able to draw a circle when shown how
- Can string large items together, such as large beads or macaroni, on a thread
- Uses a fork
- Can put some clothing on independently, like pants or a jacket

Four years:
- Holds crayons between thumb and forefinger rather than in fist
- Able to unbutton some buttons
- Can serve food and pour water (with some supervision and spilling)
- Draws a person with three or more body parts

Eye coordination[6]

Two months:
- Focuses on faces or the actions of people near them
- Eyes are not well coordinated and may appear to wander or be crossed
- Examines own hands
- Follows faces, objects, light
- Early tracking is not a smooth motion but a series of quick jumps in eye movements

Five to eight months:
- Control of eye movements and body–eye movements continues to improve, but this early tracking of an object is slow and inaccurate
- Ability to coordinate head movements with eye movements improves
- Begins to reach for objects nearby

- Recognizes familiar objects such as bottle or pacifier
- Depth perception begins to form once both eyes have the ability to coordinate together

Nine to twelve months:
- Ability to judge distance of an object improves
- Gains the ability to track faster-moving objects
- Predictive gaze tracking begins at this time, allowing a baby to anticipate where an object will go based on speed and direction
- Touches image of self in the mirror
- Crawls to reach far objects

One to two years:
- Ability to focus both near and far improves and will continue to develop until four to six years of age
- Develops clear distance vision
- Has depth perception for objects farther than two feet away
- Recognizes images of familiar objects

Two to three years:
- Improves close vision skills, convergence, and focusing
- Uses focusing to recognize shapes and objects
- Can change focus from distance to near

Hand movements in an infant begin as reflexes and then develop into consciously controlled actions through the palmar grasp reflex.[7] This reflex should be present at birth for infants and is one you've probably experienced without even realizing it. The palmar reflex is triggered when you touch a baby's hand. Your touch sends sensory information from their hand to the brain, beginning to bring awareness to their brain. The brain responds with a motor message that causes the muscles in the hand to activate and close. That's what's happening when you touch an infant's palm and they grab your finger. What feels like a sweet, bonding grasp is actually a reflex that's stimulating development in their hands by allowing the brain to process sensory input and direct the muscles to grasp. Each time this reflex is triggered, the baby is using the muscles in their hands.

Once the palmar grasp reflex has been triggered enough, the baby's brain learns to override the reflex and shifts the action of the hands from a reflex to something the child can control.

If the child doesn't fully outgrow the palmar grasp reflex, or if they never had it to begin with, they'll have less control of their hand and finger movements. When this is the case, you'll see a child using an altered pencil grasp, like using their whole fist or their thumb to help stabilize the pencil. When the reflex is still present, they have less control, so they try to stabilize their movements with that altered grasp. As a child's fine motor coordination develops, they'll write using small movements in their fingers versus large movements with their hand or arm.

Doing exercises to engage this reflex provides sensory input from the hands and builds muscle strength and coordination, contributing to the foundation of fine motor development. Stimulating this reflex enough over time allows the brain to mature beyond a reflexive movement to develop control of how the hands react to sensory input. When you understand the importance of a developmental, primitive reflex, it can help guide you in a positive direction.

When our son, Drew, was two days old, I noticed that he did *not* have the palmar grasp reflex. Getting to know my brand-new tiny baby while still in the hospital, I checked the primitive reflexes that should be present at birth. The rooting reflex, spinal galant, and other reflexes all looked good. Then I got to the palmar grasp reflex. When I touched his palm, there was no response. I checked again. And again. Then on the other side. Nada. The palmar grasp reflex wasn't present. When the next physician came in to check on us, I shared what I'd noticed. The response I got was kind but not appreciated.

"Oh, Mom, just relax and enjoy your baby boy!"

I *was* relaxed, and I was absolutely enjoying my son. But I was also aware of a piece of information that would impact Drew's development, and to me this was extremely important. Everything in development is a chain of events, so knowing he was going to be at least marginally behind in his palmar grasp reflex, I also knew he'd also most likely be behind in fine motor development and potentially speech.

I was *not* upset, and I was *not* stressed, but I now had an action plan to help Drew stay on track. All day as I was holding and snuggling Drew, I rubbed and stimulated his hands, bringing sensory awareness to them. By two months old, Drew developed the palmar grasp reflex in both hands, and over time he outgrew both reflexes.

Drew was marginally behind in speech, most notably in pronouncing his *r* sounds, and while his handwriting is still not perfect, he did win an award in third grade for his cursive writing. By acknowledging the information we had about Drew and working to put a plan in place to drive his development forward, the ramifications of his delayed reflex were extremely minor. So while that well-meaning physician blew me off, I was *happy* to know what my son needed so I could do everything I could to set him up for success.

I had another significant moment with the palmar grasp reflex one day while meeting with some parents at Brain Balance. I was describing the relevance of the palmar grasp reflex, why it was a problem that their four-year-old still had that reflex, and how that was contributing to his struggles. The dad didn't understand what I was saying, so I demonstrated how we test the reflex on him.

I first explained what it looks like in a baby—how the hand should react to the reflex with the fingers curling in to grasp the finger or object. In a toddler and beyond, when you stroke the palm of the hand there should be *no* response to the reflex stimulation. The hand should remain still even when the palm is stimulated, indicating that the brain now has control over the response and the reflex has been inhibited.

The dad placed his hands out on my desk palms up, and I leaned over and used my pen to trace a line on his palm. To my shock, the fingers on both hands curled in as if he was trying to hold my pen.

He looked at me and said, "Is this why I've never been able to type?" His wife was watching and confirmed what he said.

"He's been using a computer his whole life and still only uses his pointer fingers to type."

The dad shared that he always thought his typing and writing struggles were due to his "sausage fingers," as he called them. He was a big guy with really big fingers, but big or small fingers, you should be able to coordinate your hands to work together with ease.

The family enrolled their son in Brain Balance, and dad and son worked on the palmar grasp reflex exercises together. The son thought it was great that his dad needed to do the exercises too. I'm happy to report that both dad and son had huge gains throughout the program, and while the dad will never break any typing records, he shared that his endurance and speed were far better than they'd ever been in his life. He even picked up his old hobby of restoring a car that had been in his garage for years. With his gains in fine motor skills, working with his hands was more relaxing and enjoyable than ever before.

I experienced another developmental *aha* moment early one morning at the airport while standing in the security line. It was Christmas, and we were flying to Minnesota for the holidays. A toddler was in a stroller in line just ahead of us, and I found myself watching the child. To keep the little guy occupied, the mom handed him a book, which proved to be a great chew toy for a few minutes. Then the child was ready to engage with the book. Holding the book in his lap, he took his chubby little hand and swiped it across the cover of the book. Then he did it again. And again. Then he got mad and started to cry. The mom glanced down and quickly saw the source of his frustration. She grabbed the book and replaced it with a tablet in a childproof case. Happy now, the toddler swiped the screen, and this time the image on the screen changed. Kicking and cooing, he was happy.

The toddler knew how to operate a tablet, but he didn't know how to turn a page in the book. What the heck?! Maybe I was being dramatic—and it isn't fair to say he didn't know how to use a book after watching him for only a few minutes—but it still left a huge impression on me.

Tablets and technology are great book supplements, but they provide a different sensory experience than books do. Books have different weights and different textures to their covers and pages—there are board books, Little Golden Books, Dr. Seuss books. Each is a different shape and size. Books even have a smell. Grabbing the cover or a page to turn it (without ripping the book) requires a different set of coordination skills than swiping across a screen or tapping an object to select it.

Or maybe the child wants to tear the book and experiment with that motion, sensation, and sound, which provide even more sensory input and learning experiences. And then there's the experience of snuggling in a parent's lap and listening to the pitch and tone of their voice as they read. A variety of sensory experiences is critical to development, so be sure your kids have exposure to life outside of technology; it's crucial to their developing brain and body.

Fine Motor Development Activities for Infants and Toddlers

Refer to chapter 5 for activities that support speech and communication. In that chapter I also discuss the rooting reflex.

Fine motor skills development activities
Palmar grasp reflex

- Using a stress ball or a ball of play dough, have your child squeeze the ball, then open their hand, then squeeze again. Repeat ten to twenty times with each hand to provide sensory input to the hands and muscle activation. Next, to practice finger dexterity, have your child tap the tip of each finger with their thumb; repeat ten to twenty times with each hand. Continue to do this exercise daily for several months to build a stronger foundation for hand dexterity. For younger kids you can do this activity with your hand over theirs, gently guiding their hand to squeeze a ball and execute finger taps. Gently guide until they are able to do the activity independently, then continue for several months with the exercise.
- Have your child hang from the monkey bars. If your child is too young to do this on their own, support their body while they grip the bar. This exercises strength and sensory input to the hands.
- Create a routine of doing a quick hand massage a few times a day when you put your baby down for a nap or bedtime or while changing their diaper. Take just a moment or two to rub their palm and fingers. This touch and pressure wakes up the sensory receptors.

Beyond helping our kids develop the ability to grasp, swipe, or hold an object or device, we need to create opportunities for them to use their fingers in non-stressful scenarios to develop the feel, touch, coordination, and control that will support their interests later in life.

- Encourage sensory play with sand, bubbles, and play dough. Playing with these textures will naturally involve the child scooping up handfuls and dropping them down, squeezing the material, and experimenting with the feel on their hands. This engages sensory receptors in the brain to provide input about feel and pressure as well as works the muscles in the fingers.
- Food items are great for sensory play since infants and toddlers put nearly everything in their mouths, so incorporate them as much as possible. In fact, the hands and mouth are linked in development, so working them together is natural. Many babies have been seen sucking their thumb in utero or holding their fingers up near their mouth, so doing activities where you can use the hand and mouth together benefits both body parts as sensory perception.
- Play with peanut butter (as long as there isn't a peanut allergy), honey, Cool Whip, flour, sugar, or any other edible item that gives your child an opportunity to experience different textures, temperatures, and tastes.
- Draw with your fingers, make handprints, or even let your kids dip their fingers in honey then lick it off, which engages the mouth and hands together. You can do this during bath time or even outdoors to create a different routine. It can also make for easier cleanup after playing.
- Play toddler singing and clapping games such as "pat-a-cake, pat-a-cake, baker's man." If your child isn't able to do this on their own yet, you can provide hand-over-hand guidance and do it together to begin to engage the coordination. Remember that touch and timing engage the brain.
- As your child begins eating more table foods, allow them to feed themselves as often as possible, even when they're messy and slow.

It's a great sensory experience. Picking up the spoon, even if the applesauce gets dumped, is how they'll begin to learn to control the spoon.

Eye coordination development activities

- Keep objects within the child's range of focus (8–12 inches) to allow them to see the object, then reach and grab it
- Change the crib's position and location in their room to provide different visual input and stimuli
- Hang high-contrast visuals, such as black-and-white mobiles, within their range of viewing
- Talk to your baby while holding them; this will bring their attention to the sound of your voice and they will look to your face and exercise focusing and learning distance
- For infants five to eight months, provide mobiles and baby gym objects for them to see, touch, and pull; this will provide great fun and engagement
- For infants nine to twelve months, play peekaboo with your face and with toys to engage visual stimulation and visual memory
- Practice eye tracking with a rattle—shake the rattle to capture their attention, then slowly move the rattle within their field of vision up, down, side to side
- Roll a ball back and forth across the floor to practice eye tracking— roll the ball toward baby, away from baby, and in front of baby to practice tracking in multiple directions

Elementary School Students

Fine Motor Development Milestones
for Elementary School Students

Hands[8]

Five years:

- Writes some letters in name

Five to six years:

- Cuts out simple shapes

- Copies simple shapes like triangles
- Colors within the lines
- Uses a three-finger grasp for writing utensil
- Uses fingers to generate movement
- Pastes and glues appropriately
- Can draw basic pictures

Six to seven years:

- Forms most letters and numbers correctly
- Writes consistently on the lines
- Has good endurance for writing
- Can build with blocks, such as Lego®, independently
- Ties shoelaces independently

Seven to eight years:

- Maintains legible handwriting for an entire story

Nine to twelve years:

- Perfects and refines skills
- Handwriting becomes more fluid, automatic, and less of an effort
- Increases writing speed
- Writes well without lines

Eye coordination[9]

- Continues to improve predictive eye tracking, allowing for more accurate tracking of a moving object, with an improved ability to maintain eye contact with the target
- Quick, controlled eye movements become faster and more accurate in landing on the desired target, allowing for fast and accurate gathering of information
- Improved ability to maintain eye contact with a target, with less drifting and correcting of eye position to maintain. Gazing at an object is active, not passive, as it requires micro-adjustments in eye movements to maintain the position.
- Improved ability to correct errors in eye movements (if over-shooting a target, backs up to find target). This will continue to improve from this age until roughly fifteen years of age, when this control of eye movements should be optimized and endurance enhanced.

- Continued improvement in inhibitory actions, which stop eyes from moving to a target at the wrong time (looking at motion when you are supposed to be watching the teacher), indicating increased cognitive control. This will also continue to improve from this age until roughly fifteen years of age, when this control of eye movements should be optimized.

Six to seven years:[10]

- Readers will make small eye movements while reading, jumping two characters or less per movement
- Perceptual span indicates how much text the reader can process in one pause while reading. At this age the perceptual span is eleven characters to the right of the fixation compared to a mature reader, who can perceive fourteen or more characters to the right.

Ten to eleven years:[11]

- Readers will make much larger movements while reading, doing the small, two-character movements only 10% of the time.

Fine motor development throughout the elementary years is all about improving control, precision, and endurance. **Development continues to progress with refinement and increases in complexity as well as sequencing. Hand development progresses from gross motor movements like clapping to now being able to control two individual fingers to do something like snapping. Eye movements become faster and more accurate, and eyes can perceive more visual information. Speech now involves expressing thoughts and ideas in a logical manner.**

However, you can't build control and precision if you don't first have a solid foundation. If you've noticed any concerns in these fine motor areas, start back at the beginning of this chapter to ensure the basics are in place before working on precision and endurance.

During the pandemic, school-age kids missed out on one to two years of in-school guidance, feedback, and practice for handwriting and other fine motor skills, but we can work with them on the foundation to catch them up to age-appropriate skills.

As parents, the natural inclination is to have our kids practice what they struggle with. If their friends can tie their shoes and your child can't, you work with them over and over, hoping they'll master the task. But if they're not developmentally ready for that task, the practice becomes a hamster wheel scenario—lots of effort without progress. You wouldn't build a birdhouse without the tools. The same is true for fine motor skills and development. You first need the tools to be successful with the task.

On the topic of tools rather than practice, I made a dad angry one day. Really angry, and I didn't realize it until it was too late. This was a Brain Balance family, and the dad shared his concerns about his son's reading, focus, and fine motor skills. Chad was a great kid. He tried hard and was a people pleaser, which meant that when he struggled in school, he took it really hard. His self-confidence had tanked. He was in third grade, and his parents felt like they had a long road ahead of them in terms of school. They were already spending hours every night with Chad's homework, he was getting help in school and with a tutor, and it still wasn't enough. The parents were not ready to put him on medication, but they were starting to feel desperate.

Chad's assessment showed big areas of strength. His rhythm and timing were amazing, and his body coordination and balance were good. He also had big areas of weakness. He was still retaining several primitive reflexes, his fine motor skills were several years behind his age group, his eye tracking and coordination were behind, and his cognitive assessment confirmed that he had challenges with attention and working memory.

I felt confident we could help, and as the parents were figuring out how to work the Brain Balance schedule into their lives, I made a strong recommendation. Chad needed to focus on school and Brain Balance, and nothing else until his development was back on track. I recommended setting aside his tutor, his violin lessons, and soccer. He needed to focus on Brain Balance and also needed downtime to relax. Down the road, when his development was back on track, he could revisit soccer, violin, and the tutor and would most likely get even more out of those services at that point.

They enrolled Chad in Brain Balance, but when they left that day, his dad was upset, and I wasn't sure why. It turns out his dad was a professional violinist, and Chad had been fighting him for years over taking violin lessons. His lessons and practice didn't go well, but with all his school struggles, his dad was sure that a strong foundation in music would benefit Chad long-term. I didn't disagree; I just disagreed on the timing of the lessons. Violin requires focus, eye tracking, and fine motor skills—all areas where Chad was quite behind. It was as though they were putting a kindergartner in intense violin lessons but expecting him to play at a third-grade level. It was not a recipe for success.

The family did set aside the private violin lessons, but as a compromise, they maintained one group lesson per week for the three months Chad worked with us at Brain Balance.

About a month after completing the program, the family stopped by the office. The dad gave me a huge hug and told me he owed me a thank-you as well as an apology. He fessed up to how mad he was about the violin lessons, then told me how right I had been.

Chad had demonstrated more gains in his violin playing over the past three months—while taking a break from the weekly private lessons and daily practice—than he had demonstrated over the past several years. He now enjoyed playing the violin much more, and his teacher couldn't believe the progress that he'd made in only three months. Chad's playing improved not because he practiced but because his eyes could now track the music. He now had the focus to pay attention and the fine motor skills to manipulate the strings and bow and to read the sheet music. He was set up to succeed as a violinist. I'm not sure Chad will ever become a professional musician like his dad, but he got to a point where he both enjoyed playing and felt successful doing it.

The violin teacher reached out to ask if there were any exercises he could do with his other students to help their fine motor skills for hands and eyes improve the way they had for Chad. While it isn't possible to re-create the Brain Balance program on your own, as it involves many proprietary software technologies, gear, and protocols, there are effective activities you can do on your own to benefit development. I provided him with two palmar grasp exercises his students could do as a warm-up to facilitate their finger dexterity. (Details on these exercises can be found earlier in this chapter.) The first exercise involves holding a soft ball in the palm of your hand and simply squeezing the ball, then opening your hand and squeezing again. Each time the ball is squeezed the hand is receiving sensory input, and the nerves and muscles that control the hands are engaged. The second exercise has students do finger taps to tap each finger with the thumb. This detailed task again works the nerves and muscles and requires patience and control to align the tip of each finger with the thumb to tap it.

Progress in fine motor skills at this age comes from a solid foundation, then exposure, experimentation, and practice. Building new pathways and strengthening existing pathways in the brain requires repetition. Think of this like "muscle memory" where you can do a physical coordination task without thought. You've practiced the pattern to a point that your body does what it needs to do with little effort. Tying your shoes started as an arduous process that over time became something you could do while completely distracted by other things. This is an example of strong and efficient pathways that can be used with ease.

Fine Motor Development Activities for Elementary School Students

Palmar grasp reflex
- Squeeze and release a ball; repeat
- Tap each finger to the thumb, making sure the tips of the fingers are touching, until you are able to do this quickly and easily in both directions, while using both hands at the same time

Grip strength and sensory input
- Play on the monkey bars
- Work on batting practice (holding the bat, feeling the vibration when you hit the ball)
- Practice the golf club grip; this is a different grip from that for a baseball bat, and it's a different feel when you swing the club and hit the ball
- Learn to snap your fingers

Arts, crafts, and hobbies to develop fine motor skills
- Paint, draw, color

- Work with clay, play dough, pottery
- Build something with a hammer and nails (and supervision)—a birdhouse or book shelf
- Bake cookies, roll out cookie dough, cut out cookies
- Decorate cookies or a cake
- Make bead necklaces or knotted friendship bracelets
- Knit or crochet a blanket
- Play dominoes, jacks, Jenga
- Play with Lego® blocks, model airplanes, or rockets
- Learn the alphabet and words in sign language
- Learn cursive or calligraphy
- Build your own computer or robot

Middle School and High School Students

School at this age is less about cutting and pasting for art class and more about cramming in content, papers, and projects—all of which are still heavily dependent on the complexity of coordinating small movements and muscles: eye tracking to read, the hands to type and take notes, and the mouth and tongue to express thoughts and opinions through speech.

Fine Motor Development Milestones for
Middle School and High School Students

Beyond age fourteen, fine motor development is not expected to continue to improve in developmental coordination without specific practice and exercise, such as training or repetition for a sport or hobby. This means that your foundational skills are expected to be set at this point, yet you can still improve through effort and practice. What continue to improve at this age are impulse control and executive functions, which result in better focus in the face of distractions and improved planning and execution when working to achieve goals. This impacts how a student takes notes in class, that is, their ability to write in shorthand to summarize what the teacher is saying. Continued improvement for eye movements means the increased ability to block out visual distractions—the student gets better at overriding the impulse to shift their eyes to look at movement when in class. And for speech this involves clear articulation of thoughts and ideas, and the impulse control to keep some thoughts to themselves.

Our teens were already using technology in school when the pandemic hit, then shifted to using even more technology. They had more time on tablets and phones, using their fingers to swipe, tap, or scribble out math problems. They spent more time on computers, typing their answers and submitting assignments with screenshots and attachments. And they had more unsupervised time with even more access to tech than ever before—which sharply curtailed the variety in how kids entertained themselves as the months stretched into years.

Recent research is starting to uncover the impact these changes have had on the visual systems for kids during this time. A study out of Hong Kong and published in the *British Journal of Ophthalmology* involving over 1,700 students found a steep increase in rates of myopia—nearsightedness—during the pandemic, attributed to less time spent outdoors and more time spent on devices.[12] Additional studies found increased rates of kids struggling with vergence—the ability for the eyes to work together to keep an object clear in sight whether the object is near or far. Also noted were increases in visual fatigue and dry eyes.[13]

Increased tech time, and decreased time exercising the eyes as they shift from the teacher to the paper and back again, took a toll, and while glasses can help how clearly you see at a distance, glasses are not the answer for all visual system challenges. Like your body, the eyes are also controlled by nerves and muscles and need to fire with perfect timing to accomplish a motor task successfully—and they require exercise and activation to remain in prime shape. You can't assume that just because your child is in high school that their fine motor skills are maximized.

When it comes to development, keep in mind that your child's actual age and their level of development in a particular category may not always align. Zach was a prime example of someone whose chronological age was misaligned with his fine motor development. His mom reached out for an exploratory conversation, not sure where to turn for help. While Zach had areas of struggle, he didn't have a formal diagnosis or label. His mom shared that he'd never fit neatly into any one category.

Zach got along well with others and didn't have a behavior problem at school or at home, but while he had friends, he at times seemed younger than his peers. This was especially noticeable if he was frustrated or upset. School was a struggle, and while he enjoyed sports, he wasn't overly athletic. His parents felt like they'd never been able to truly pinpoint or address what was going on, but deep down his mom felt there was more to Zach and wanted to figure out how to support him. When Zach was young, they had spent time in speech and occupational therapy, eventually graduating out of those services. His parents felt like they'd run out of options and didn't know what else they could do to support their son. Could Brain Balance help? Since they didn't live near a Brain Balance center, they did the Brain Balance home program, working with a live coach via computer each week to guide them.

When he started the program, Zach was behind in some, but not all, areas, most notably his auditory and visual processing, fine motor skills, and eye movements involved in reading and shifting from near to far. His eyes would overshoot or undershoot the target, resulting in many increased eye movements for each line of text he read. He had his work cut out for him.

Zach was quiet during the sessions but was cooperative and worked hard, and his mom said she felt like everything he was doing was good for him. She was also pleased with how different the exercises and activities were from other things they'd tried in the past. She was cautiously optimistic.

About two months into the program, Zach's dad left a voicemail. In fact, he called twice. When he left the message the first time, he got so excited he hung up and had to call back a second time to share his story.

Zach had asked for a pair of high-top Air Jordans, the popular shoes at school. His parents automatically said no, since at fourteen, Zach still wasn't able to tie his shoes. Zach kept pushing, and eventually his mom relented. He said he'd be willing to try once more to tie his shoes if they'd spend the money to get these fancy sneakers. His mom was dreading this, as over and over it had ended it tears and frustration—sometimes for both of them. With high-tops, he'd have to tie and untie these shoes every time he wore them, and his parents wouldn't always be around to help out if needed.

His dad got home from work that day and was greeted by Zach wearing his new shoes, grinning from ear to ear. He had tied his own shoes for the first time ever. His mom confirmed that she'd showed him how to do it one time, and after that, he completely got it on his own.

On the voicemail, the dad said, "I know it doesn't sound like a big deal for a fourteen-year-old to tie their own shoes. But what you don't understand is that he was fourteen and *still* couldn't tie his shoes, and it wasn't from lack of trying. For eight years we tried to teach him over and over, and nothing worked. It meant so much to see that smile on Zach's face, knowing that it was a smile of pride."

Over the course of the program, they continued to see gains in Zach's reading and school work, as well as his confidence and willingness to speak up and become more involved in class. He was handling himself so much better when he got frustrated and seemed much more age appropriate in his behaviors. He was a happy kid whose confidence continued to grow as he felt more successful in what he was doing at school and at home—and in the trendy shoes he could wear like the other kids. For Zach, the time during the pandemic gave his family a chance to focus on the elements of his development that needed help, allowing his functions to spring forward during that crazy time.

Zach needed strengthening in auditory and visual pathways as well as in timing and coordination. The next step in order for Zach to continue to see gains is practice and play. His functionals have improved so much, and now is the time to try new activities, or activities that may have been hard in the past. To continue to push and grow he needs to put those functions into practice—so they continue to improve in their ease and efficiency.

One of my favorite parenting mantras, much to the chagrin of my children, is *boredom sparks creativity.* We spend so much of our lives actively engaged in something: work, school, technology. We leave very little time in our lives for free thinking and creativity. When kids aren't told what to do and they aren't engrossed in their devices, that's when creativity and growth continue to happen—at every age. You are never too old to play.

Years ago, when going to the beach for a week, we got in the habit of not using our devices, and it's a habit we've tried to maintain over the years. Instead of scrolling TikTok and YouTube, the kids are out exploring: catching blue crabs by tying chicken wings to a string and dropping them over the edge of a dock in the salt marshes, throwing out the cast net for bait fish, or casting out a line to try to catch something. They are playing, and through play they're refining their fine motor skills, receiving varied sensory input, and practicing coordination and timing, while letting their thoughts and mind wander. Without the constant distraction of technology, the kids still manage to stay active and busy, even though it is an entire chunk of unstructured time.

Fine Motor Development Activities for Middle School and High School Students

Use all the suggestions from the elementary-aged kids as well as the following:

Grip strength and sensory input
- Use a pull-up bar to work on upper body strength and hand strength
- Play tennis or pickleball
- Cook or bake
  - Make your own sushi rolls
  - Bake bread, kneading the dough and rolling it out
  - Have a cake decorating contest with friends
  - Make homemade cannoli
  - Dice fruit to make a smoothie
  - Host a fondue night with friends. Chop a variety of snacks and treats to dip into melted cheese or chocolate
- Enjoy arts, crafts, and hobbies
  - Go for a hike and collect leaves and flowers to arrange in a vase to decorate your room
  - Paint designs on your fingernails and toenails
  - Make your own set of thank-you cards or a scrapbook
  - Take apart and rebuild something (with parental permission, of course!)

Eye coordination
- Shift eyes from near to a mid-distance to far and back again (great practice and prep for driving to be able to quickly glance from the

road, to the dashboard, and back up again). You can do this anywhere. Simply look at something 12–18 inches in front of you, then without shifting your head quickly look up and focus on something farther away, then again on something farther in the distance. Return your eyes to the midpoint, then to the near point. Shift back and forth as quickly as you can while still focusing on each object clearly before shifting. You can use your thumbs and a wall to do this. Hold one thumb in a "thumbs up" position approximately one foot in front of your nose. Extend out your other arm with that thumb in the same position. Now shift your eyes from your close thumb, to the far thumb, to the wall, and back.

- Practice quick, targeted eye movements. Hold your two thumbs up about a foot apart. Quickly shift your eyes back and forth between the thumbs with the goal of landing exactly on your thumbnail and moving as fast as you can. Repeat ten times. Then shift positions and repeat. Each time you do this exercise you can shift the position in which you hold your thumbs to move your eyes in different directions.

Signs That Indicate Improvement

As toddlers mature in their finger dexterity fine motor skills, you'll notice a shift in the toys and activities that interest them. They'll seek out smaller objects as they become more adept with their hands and will shift from playing with larger to smaller blocks, cars, and toys. They'll also show more interest in coloring.

In kids who are a little older, you'll begin to notice a change in their coloring and drawing skills. It will begin with a greater interest in coloring, and they'll start to engage in the task for longer periods of time as it becomes more fun and less frustrating. About this same time, you'll notice their improved ability to feed themselves, with marginally less food ending up on the floor or in their hair. They'll become more adept at picking up one morsel of food at a time rather than using their entire hand to grab whatever they can. Navigating the spoon from the bowl to their mouth will improve, and they'll begin using a fork successfully.

For kids who are able to write, you'll know their fine motor skills are improving when you notice a change in the amount of pressure they apply when writing—it will either become less or more. Their letter shape, size, and spacing will become more consistent, as will the letters and numbers themselves.

About this time, you may notice them shift from using their entire arm to write and draw to moving only their hands and fingers.

As older kids experience gains in fine motor skills, you should begin to notice less complaining about writing tasks, less hand cramping, and less task avoidance, because the physical act of writing has become less of a chore.

As speech fine motor skills improve, your child will speak more, even if they are older. You will notice more sounds, more words, longer sentences, and more involved stories. Thoughts will be told in the correct sequence, so you can follow along and understand. The stronger and more efficient these pathways become, the less energy they will take—so even if your child is tired after a long day at school, you just may get more than a one-word answer.

When eye coordination and endurance improve, reading and keeping up in class become easier. Less energy and effort will be needed to slug through a passage, which leaves more energy for paying attention to the content and remembering what was read.

4

. . . .

ATTENTION

" **P**ay attention, hold still, try harder, you can do this. Keep your hands to yourself. STOP! Listen. How many times do I have to repeat myself? Focus!"

Sound familiar? If you've ever said this to your kids, please read this chapter carefully. It's a heavy one, but it's important.

If you've noticed your kids—or even yourself—feeling distracted, stressed, overwhelmed, emotional, or burned out, you're not alone. You may also have noticed they have challenges with staying on task, doing the work, *and* turning it in, or inconsistencies in behavior and work. These are all indicators of disruptions in focus.

During the pandemic, rates of childhood and adult attention deficit hyperactivity disorder (ADHD), depression, and anxiety increased. In fact, research has shown that the pandemic exacerbated the core issues of ADHD.[1] And it's important to note that your child does not need a diagnosis to struggle. **Focus, motivation, mood management, organization, task completion—all get harder when you're stressed or overwhelmed—whether you have ADHD or not. If you do have ADHD, stress and fatigue will amplify those challenges, making everything an even steeper uphill climb.**

Note to Parents

Most people are familiar with the stereotypical ADHD boy, the hyperactive eight-year-old falling out of his chair at school, and while this can be true, attention challenges don't always present this obviously. Disruptions in attention can be loud and impulsive, but this isn't always the case, making attentional concerns easier to miss and harder to support. It's important to note that immaturity in attention can look different in adults than in kids, and in males versus females. The concerns of attention can be quiet and subtle in both their symptoms and effects. When attention is low, you may see an uptick in anxiety. There may be errors and mistakes more frequently. There may be inconsistency in the level and quality of work. Feelings of self-doubt, shame, and inadequacy may arise. There might be more procrastination, and even a perfectionism mindset. Challenges controlling temper and bigger reactions to life's frustrations may occur. Losing one's temper or control can then amplify those feelings of shame to the point where the person struggling may ask, "What's wrong with me? Why can everyone else do this, and it's hard for me?"

Many studies have been done to understand the full scope of ADHD. The list of heightened concerns is long. Children with ADHD have been shown to have increased difficulties in school, including academic underperformance (where your child's quality of work and testing doesn't align with their intelligence and abilities), and struggles with relationships with peers and family. They are at more risk for both bullying and being bullied, as well as conduct and behavioral challenges, including oppositional defiant disorder and antisocial behaviors. There is a higher risk for substance use and abuse. There are also higher rates of mental well-being concerns, including depression, anxiety, and low self-esteem.[2]

It's also important to note you don't need an official diagnosis of ADHD for disruptions in attention to be negatively impacting many areas of life. Subthreshold ADHD means challenges are present but fall just shy of meeting the diagnostic criteria. While subthreshold ADHD is rarely discussed, it impacts nearly twice as many as those with a known diagnosis. The pre-pandemic rate of ADHD in kids was roughly 10%, with an estimated 17% of additional kids experiencing subthreshold ADHD.[3] This means that one in four kids have aspects of their attentional systems impacting their daily lives. Challenges with attention make executing complex tasks and regulating your mood and behavior more difficult, requiring more energy and effort, which fatigues the brain. Prolonged states of stress contribute to fatigue as well. Combining a lack of attention with higher levels of stress and fatigue creates a big uphill battle. So if you've noticed your kids are distracted, require reminders to stay on task or turn in work, or feel overwhelmed, negative, or frustrated, it could be related to the development of their attentional systems and may be further exacerbated by what is happening in life.

Understanding how attention develops in the brain and the role sensory perception plays, as well as the various nuances of attention, can equip you with an opportunity to make things better in times of both stress and calm. The concepts that support improving attention in your kids can also have a positive impact on *your* brain, helping to boost mood, focus, and productivity.

Pandemic Lessons

The pandemic brought challenge after challenge to our attentional abilities. STRESS. Check. CHANGE. Check. DISTRACTIONS (the entire family doing work and school from home). Check. TASK-SWITCHING (supervising the entire family forced us to multi-task more than ever). Check.

In addition to all the competition for our attention, we had increased time on devices and less physical activity.[4] We decreased what energizes the brain (exercise) and increased what drains the brain (tons of screen time). With that combination, we were given an incredibly powerful reminder of the importance of how development and daily life impact the success of our attentional networks.

The pandemic created the perfect storm to crush our attention, which is reflected in the data: more people now face attention and ADHD challenges than before, with a sharp increase in ADHD diagnoses.[5] Seventeen percent more kids started meds during the pandemic than in the previous year (2019), and even more changed, added, or adjusted their current medication use. And for those already diagnosed with ADHD, challenges and symptoms increased.[6]

The pandemic period showed us how susceptible our attention is to both our activities and levels of stress. Now we can leverage those lessons to enhance attention!

Science Alert

Attention. It's one word that we use to describe many different things. Like the weather, attention is always there, but it has many variations with differing, but necessary, purposes. While we all enjoy some elements of the weather more than others, we can agree that sun, rain, and wind are all necessary. Attention also has different aspects that are necessary and serve various purposes, but, unlike with the weather, you have the ability to impact and even change your attentional abilities.

Attention refers to how we engage and interact with the world, and it's how our brain prioritizes information. We can't possibly process or store all the information and stimuli that happen around us, so, like the reticular activating system (RAS) we discussed previously, our attention acts as another form of gatekeeper to control what information we collect and store. Attention blocks the brain from having to take in too much since we can't possibly store it all. But this gatekeeper storage system is not the same in all people—or for all ages.

Over time, through development and demand, our attentional systems mature and improve by optimizing neural networks. These networks and regions of the brain require fuel to do their job. Optimized, or mature neural networks, fire with greater speed and efficiency, requiring less fuel to function. Using less fuel allows the networks supporting the attentional systems to perform longer before fatiguing, which in turn allows us to stay on task longer, better control impulses, and block out distractions. But the attentional system is not the only region in the brain requiring fuel; this resource is shared with other regions and functions. High levels of stress or fatigue or sensory input are all examples of what will also drain fuel reserves. The sharing of resources throughout the brain is why the same person may not have consistent attentional abilities day in and day out. Each day we're faced with different levels of demands, distractions, and energy, which can chip away at our ability to perform at our best.

Attention is a fascinating topic that could easily fill an entire book, but since everyone doesn't find the topic as exciting as I do, I'll narrow it down to a few key elements. To understand how to enhance and support attention, I'll touch on four topics: environmental attention, focused attention, what competes with your ability to focus, and fuel.

The first thing to realize is that while we often yell at our kids to "pay attention!" we're all paying attention. All the time. What differs is the *type* of attention we use in the moment.

I describe the first type of attention as *environmental attention*. This type of attention is broad and general. It allows us to sweep the environment to be aware of what's happening around us in a relaxed and generalized manner. Picture driving down the highway on a long road trip. You're watching the road while your mind wanders. You won't remember much of what you see, or your thoughts, but you're paying enough attention to kick into high gear if necessary. When this type of attention is triggered, you aren't actively engaged in a task that requires thought or large amounts of effort, and your mind is able to wander from topic to topic. You can maintain this state of attention for long periods of time, since it requires almost no effort or fuel to support. This is also the type of attention that kicks in when you're reading and you glaze over. Your eyes are going through the motions, but you aren't engaging with the content. (Fingers crossed that isn't happening to you now.)

The scientific name for the parts of the brain involved in this environmental attention is the *default mode network*. It's a set of pathways in the brain that involves multiple brain regions that are more active during passive tasks than during activities that require focused attention. It's what contributes to your mind wandering, as well as thinking about the future and remembering things from the past.[7] Dr. Amishi Jha, an attention researcher and the author of *Peak Mind: Find Your Focus, Own Your Attention, Invest 12 Minutes a Day*, relates this type of attention to a floodlight. We are aware of anything the bright light shines on.[8]

When our attention is in an environmental state, it's scanning our environment to keep us safe in the world. Our thoughts will scan not only our surroundings, but also the past and the future and can often result in stress and worries. *Do I have enough time today to get the groceries, laundry, and all my writing done? Did I remember to answer that email from last week?* For some people, this can be an uncomfortable state, as it can generate worries about upcoming events or memories from the past. That person may find themselves reaching for their phone or other distractions as a way to change their focus to actively engage their brain and disrupt their own thoughts.

The default mode network provides us many positive benefits. This jumping of thoughts and memories helps us process emotions and events, allows us to daydream and brainstorm, and contributes to our creativity.

Research has shown that for individuals with ADHD, the default network has atypical connectivity and is more active than in those without ADHD.[9] This means that someone with ADHD is more likely to experience mind wandering and, since their environmental attention is active more frequently, more likely to worry about the future and the past.

The next type of attention is *focused attention*. This aspect of attention is what we think of when we say, "Pay attention! Are you listening to me?" Focused attention is the ability to respond to specific stimuli—auditory, visual, or tactile—and then bring selective information to the brain and into your awareness.[10]

An example of focused attention would be a child sitting in the classroom who's zeroed in on the teacher. Focused attention will *not* be alerting the brain to other environmental stimuli—such as the other wiggly kids in the classroom—but will relay the information the brain thinks is relevant to what the child is trying to learn. Focused attention creates the ability to listen and take notes from what the teacher is saying to be prepared for the test. There's a higher likelihood of retaining information that makes it to the brain when using focused attention, but this type of attention requires more fuel to support the brain than environmental attention does.

The goal is to be able to maintain focused attention long enough to complete the task at hand. The *Encyclopedia of Neuropsychology* describes this type of attention as maintaining vigilance or alertness over time. This sustained attention is considered a fundamental component of your cognitive abilities.[11] You can't learn or remember if you can't pay attention.

Focused attention requires more pathways and whole-brain connections (which result from development) to override distractions and impulses. This brain function has high fuel needs to support these pathways. Thus, your ability to sustain focused attention is related to your development and available fuel, and it is harder to maintain this aspect of attention for long.

When the brain runs low on fuel, is on overload, or becomes distracted by other stimuli, it will shift back into environmental attention, which requires minimal fuel to function but results in the mind wandering and less retention of what the teacher is saying.

Like many parents, you may be wondering how the attention needed for gaming or social media fits into this discussion. Every parent I know at some point has asked a question along the lines of, "How is it that my child can focus for hours of video games but can't sit still for 20 minutes of math?" The answer is a critical nuance to understanding your child's attention.

The attention used to watch TikTok videos or gaming is not utilizing two hours of the type of focused attention we just discussed but is using microbursts of attention strung together because of the reward system in the brain. These microbursts of attention are laser-focused on the task at hand, helping you achieve your goal. In this period, you are unaware of your surroundings and disconnect from your awareness of time. This allows you to take a break from any stressors or worries in life you may be facing. Then when you achieve your goal—points or the next level in the video game, or a laugh while watching a funny video—the brain rewards you by releasing dopamine, a feel-good neurochemical. To earn more rewards, more dopamine, the brain re-engages in the next microburst of attention. **Two hours of gaming is not two hours of focused attention but hundreds of microbursts of attention strung together by a reward to fill two hours.**

Microbursts of attention come at a high cost for fuel needs, depleting the tank. Which is why you're often faced with very negative kids and behaviors after hours spent gaming. When they stop gaming, and the dopamine reward that re-engaged their attention goes away, their mood and energy crash. They aren't throwing a fit just because they don't want to stop, but also because they have run out of the fuel needed to control their actions and behaviors.

The focused attention driven by rewards is powerful and necessary in achieving our goals but isn't the aspect of focused attention needed to succeed in school and work. Most of our lives require long periods of focused attention, with very little reward.

Remember, the brain pathways we use are the ones we strengthen. When our kids spend hours each day on their devices, they are strengthening their reward-driven pathways and behaviors. Our kids will benefit from more time spent exercising sustained focus than reward-driven focus.

It's interesting to note that video game developers are very aware of this fact and build this concept into their games to keep you actively engaged for longer periods of time. There was even a lawsuit by parents whose two kids became addicted to a game. The parents sued the gaming company Epic Games for "knowingly making an addictive game that was designed to cause the release of dopamine in the players' brains similar to that caused by drugs like cocaine, which can ultimately lead to a chemical addiction."[12] While nothing appeared to come from the lawsuit as of early 2023, it demonstrates the awareness of the reward-driven pathways, which are different from the attentional pathways needed for school.

Environmental attention, focused attention, and microbursts of attention are all utilized throughout each day. We toggle back and forth between the different elements of attention without even realizing it. Having a better understanding of attention can help both you and your child become more self-aware and plan ways to support the type of attention that is needed for a goal or task.

Due to the complexity of our attentional systems, many factors can interfere with our attention. Understanding what competes with or minimizes our attention is the next step to optimizing attentional performance. Immaturities in development result in pathways that are less efficient, making it harder to pay attention for long periods of time and harder to override impulses and block out distractions. Change, stress, task-switching, distractions, and development are all also elements that impact attention, as is the fuel needed to support this function.

- Change: An article titled "We Are Hardwired to Resist Change" by Chris Pennington, a business consulting manager, discusses that the amygdala, the emotional center of the brain, perceives change as an unknown or a threat and releases stress hormones in response.[13] This can even be uncomfortable for many people. It requires you to expend more intentional energy and effort, to spend more time in sustained focus while experiencing stress hormones that wear you down. Facing change is like running uphill on a day you're exhausted. Your daily habits require little effort, but to actively work to break those habituations requires a lot of effort. This focus and effort drain precious resources, and a brain that runs out of fuel will become tired, irritable, negative, and more likely to revert to old habits. For example, trying to cut down on social media usage. When you're focused on your goal, you can stay on task, but when you become tired, stressed, or distracted, it's easy to forget the goal and revert to the habit—like checking your phone when you're stuck in traffic. Keeping the goal top-of-mind is necessary and requires additional reminders, fuel, and focused attention to accomplish.

- Stress: Stress also drains and challenges the brain, but in a different way than change, although both can deplete fuel (in chapters 7 and 8 we'll do a deeper dive to understand stress). Stress puts the brain on high alert and prepares you to be ready for anything. It delivers heightened focus and awareness of your environment. Stress also sends your thoughts racing in many directions—and it's human nature to think through worst-case scenarios. Worrying about everything that could go wrong or being stuck in a memory where you encountered similar stress are reactions that play out in the brain.[14] You can't maintain this state for long, and when you crash, you'll be exhausted.

- Task-switching: While our culture celebrates multi-tasking, it's a major factor that detracts from our ability to optimize sustained attention. Our brain has a hard time doing multiple things at the same time. Instead, we tend to bounce back and forth between tasks to multi-task. Making dinner while checking email? You can't actually focus on both at the same time, and each time you stop reading your email to stir the pot, your focus shifts from the email topic to dinner. Remember that focused attention is a finite thing. It doesn't last forever, and each time you pull your focus from one task to address another, you quickly drain your resources. If you stop to read or respond each time the computer dings for an incoming message or your phone vibrates with a text, you've lost an opportunity to focus for longer. It's a better strategy to work on a single task at a time for things that require more thought and effort to accomplish. We need to teach our kids to create a habit of single-task focusing because it will serve them well going forward.

- Distractions: Distractions create accidental task-switching moments. Imagine your son is in the kitchen doing math homework. Every time someone walks into the kitchen, he looks up to see what they're doing. Each time is a missed opportunity for sustained focus. Distractions often come from sensory input—a noise that startles you, a person that bumps into you, or something that moves in your peripheral vision, so you look up to check it out. Wherever your eyes look, that's where your attention is focused. A brain that processes sensory input well is more able to block out distracting input, but a brain that perceives this input as *amplified compared to how others perceive it* will be more susceptible to distractions and will fatigue more quickly.

- Development: Attention is something that evolves in control and duration over time and is highly dependent on impulse control. A two-year-old spends just a few minutes at a time in focused attention before wandering off to explore the next thing that captures their interest. A five-year-old can sit for longer during circle time in kindergarten while singing songs and talking about the weather and the days of the week. A ten-year-old can work independently in class—or at home—for homework. An adult can toil away all day at work. As the networks and pathways in our brain become faster, more efficient, and more complex, we improve our ability to choose how to direct our attention, block out distractions, resist impulses, and sustain our attention for longer. Any disruptions in development can also impact our attentional skills and abilities.[15]

- Fuel: Like a car, the brain can't run without fuel, and that fuel comes from the foods we eat. Different activities burn fuel at different rates. So, while half a tank of gas may allow you to do your math homework, you may need a full tank to do that homework, then turn your attention to science—while maintaining a positive mood. There are entire books dedicated to eating for brain health, but here are a few quick takeaways:

1. The brain and body require an array of nutrients. It's critical to consume a variety of foods to provide all the necessary elements. If your child is a picky eater, understanding which nutrients they are *not* consuming is important so you can find high-quality supplements to address any nutrition gaps. While my preference is to always address nutritional needs through food, supplementing for the gaps is better than not addressing the gaps at all.

2. Not all fuel burns at the same rate. Sugar provides energy but burns out quickly, while protein and healthy fats are fuel sources that burn more slowly, providing fuel for longer periods of time. Ensuring your kids are eating protein in addition to carbohydrates consistently throughout the day can help to support sustained focus, mood, and energy while minimizing the peaks and crashes that result in tantrums and upsets. Kids (and adults) love treats, and that's okay. Having a "fuel first" mentality when it comes to eating allows you to still enjoy the treats, but only after you've given your body what it needs to be strong, healthy, and focused.

Infants and Toddlers

While we don't typically think about a baby's attention, these foundational elements begin to lay the groundwork for future abilities. Processing sensory input to understand what is happening in the environment and eye tracking to guide *where* to direct attention start from the very beginning.

Note that developmental expectations and attention milestones aren't mapped out for infants until eighteen months of age.

Attention Development Milestones for Infants and Toddlers

Eighteen months:[16]
- Will look at a few pages in a book with you

Two years:[17]
- Four to six minutes of sustained attention

Four years:[18]

- Eight to twelve minutes of sustained attention

To begin to better understand your child's attentional abilities, the best place to start is with simple observation. Watching your toddler will show you interesting nuances regarding their attention. When they're engaged with something they love, how long do they remain on-task when they're playing on their own? If you're working with them on something such as learning colors, what do their attention and behavior look like? How long do they remain engaged? What pulls their attention and what holds their attention?

Take notes and use this information as just that—information. Not a judgment but a benchmark to use to track growth and progress. Set your expectations based on what your child can do right now, not based on the developmental milestone expectation. (You can use that information to see how your child is tracking, and if they're behind, focusing on the foundational aspects of coordination and sensory development will help to get their attentional abilities back on track.)

Once you have a better sense of their current attentional abilities, honor it. Don't set expectations higher than their current abilities. If their sustained attention is two minutes, don't try to push it to five minutes. That time will not be productive and will leave you both feeling frustrated. Instead, maximize those two minutes by creating an environment of minimal distraction and have everything prepared for what you want to do, so you aren't wasting time looking for a certain book or toy. Plan this two-minute window of focus for when your child is rested and fed, since fatigue and hunger will disrupt attention.

During your window of focused time, engage their senses to help hold their attention and to connect multiple pathways and regions of their brain. If you are looking at the color red, find something they can look at, touch, smell, and even taste that is red. Once those two minutes are up, give your child a break. Let them wander over to whatever captures their interest next. (Movement rather than technology will be a more effective strategy to give them a break if you want them to re-engage.)

Honoring the child's window of focus and carefully choosing the time made a big difference in bedtime for a friend of mine. She knew that it was good to create a bedtime routine, and as a working mom, this was the best time in her day to set everything aside to focus on her little girl. Bath time, reading books, learning, and talking about the day were all part of their routine.

On a walk together one evening, my friend shared a concern with me that she'd been harboring for several months.

"I know she's smart, but I worry about her learning and how she'll do in school."

When I asked why she was so worried when Ella was only three, she said that her daughter wouldn't focus and had no interest in learning things like shapes and colors. It was like they started over from scratch every day, and it wasn't unusual for Ella to get angry or cry rather than cooperate. Since they weren't sending Ella to preschool during the pandemic, she felt extra pressure to ensure they taught the basics at home, so Ella wouldn't be behind when school started.

After asking a few more questions, I felt confident that the answer had little to do with Ella's abilities to learn and more to do with my friend's timing and expectations. Their bedtime routine took an hour, and the learning time came *after* a bath and reading several books—right before prayers and sleep. My friend was asking her three-year-old to focus and learn when she was exhausted. I encouraged her to flip the routine to a time when Ella was rested and before doing anything else that required focus.

My friend called a few weeks later with good news to report. She started getting up fifteen minutes earlier and switched their learning time to the morning. After Ella was fed and dressed, they took a few short minutes to do their "work." Within just a week, Ella had learned and retained more colors and shapes than in the past few months combined. The issue was the timing and parent expectations (which were too long for a three-year-old), not her abilities.

After you've observed your child's attentional abilities, intentional practice becomes helpful. Remember, the more you use the pathways in the brain, the faster, stronger, and more efficient those pathways become. Use that two-minute window of attention (or however long it is for your child) multiple times throughout the day. Remember that this type of attention is not based on a dopamine reward from the brain, so there's no need to celebrate the moment when it's done. Simply use the time to practice sustained attention. You can read a book, color a picture, talk about something you see out the window, sing a song—any activity that engages your toddler so their thoughts and mind aren't wandering will exercise their sustained, focused attention.

Beyond observing your child to determine their window of attentional abilities and sustained attention, you may also notice clues that indicate whether your child's attention is being impacted by a startle stimulus. If you've noticed your child becoming upset over loud noises such as fireworks or the vacuum cleaner, there may be more going on that's disrupting their attention than simply over-processing noise. Kids who retain the startle reflex may also be more prone to frustrations and meltdowns and more easily distracted.[19] An over-reactive startle reaction can be related to another primitive reflex called the *Moro reflex*. Babies should be born with this reflex, like other reflexes, then eventually outgrow it by six months, resulting in greater control over their reactions.[20] This reflex is described as an involuntary protective motor response that's triggered through body disruption or strong stimuli. That strong stimuli can include touch, sound, or even a change in lighting, as well as a change in body position or balance. The motor response is an extension response. The head will shift back, and the arms and legs will move outward, then curl back in again.[21] Long before we knew what this was, my husband and I observed this reflex in our infant daughter. We were eating dinner one night, and Morgan was sleeping in the bouncy seat at our feet. Doug was telling a story and, per his usual self, was quite animated, clapping his hands loudly at one point. When he clapped, Morgan's hands popped up, her fingers splayed wide, then relaxed back into position resting on her chest—all without her waking up.

"Did you see that?" Doug asked.

He clapped his hands again to see what would happen, and sure enough, the same response occurred. I also noticed the same response when I tried to transition from holding her in my arms to laying her down in the crib.

Unless she was swaddled tightly and I laid her down just so, that transition would trigger her to jump and make those little arms pop up, which would wake her up and start the process of trying to get her asleep in her crib all over again.

While you're supposed to have this reaction as an infant, you shouldn't have it as a toddler, child, or adult. Imagine how you'd react when startled. You're sitting in your office working at the computer when suddenly the front door closes with a bang. You react with a gasp and shout, "What was that?" You're now on high alert, listening for clues about what just happened and wondering if everything is okay. When you realize it was just the wind, and everyone's fine, you shift your focus back to your work. But that startle stimulus pulled your attention and triggered a response that accelerated your heart rate and breathing, caused pupil dilation, and impacted your thoughts and mood.

When a startle stimulus is big enough, we *should* all react; however, for people who have not outgrown the infant Moro reflex, their body responds to small stimuli as though it was a much bigger prompt. Can you image how stressed and fatigued you'd feel if an unexpected noise or touch triggered your "what was that?!" response all day long? You'd struggle much more to maintain focused attention, and you'd be more irritable. In fact, studies have shown that retaining primitive reflexes, including the Moro reflex, is associated with attentional problems in school-aged children[22] and motor problems in preschool-aged children[23] and may predict later development of anxiety and depression.[24]

Marco was a four-year-old who came to see us at Brain Balance. He was the youngest of five kids, so his parents had lots of experience with what development looked like for a child this age in terms of behavior and attention. His mom said that his teacher's main concern was Marco's lack of attention, and the teacher had brought it up to her on several occasions. While she agreed that his attention was a problem, she was also very concerned about his anxiety. She felt it was holding him back from engaging with other kids and activities.

Marco was the kid who would cling to her leg at drop-off and was hesitant to engage with other kids. Because Marco struggled to get comfortable with anything new or different, his parents kept him enrolled in preschool as much as they could throughout the pandemic. His behavior wasn't loud or disruptive, but he would wander off and wouldn't engage in circle time or activities for long.

After starting the Brain Balance program, his parents knew big changes were happening with Marco's attention and anxiety when the playground helper commented on the differences she'd noticed in him. She had no idea they were doing anything to support Marco. She just wanted to share the growth and change she'd noticed. Marco was now running around and playing with the other kids and even initiating interactions. His classroom teacher confirmed those changes and also shared that Marco was able to stay seated for circle times on most days (not perfect, but progress). He no longer cried after parent drop-off, and he was speaking up more in class.

While Marco experienced growth in all areas at Brain Balance, one of the biggest changes for him was that his startle reflex went from being severe to inhibited. This allowed his body to be more relaxed, calm, and present rather than constantly distracted and overreacting to the world around him. (When I ran into Marco's mom years later, she shared that after the program he had continued to grow and thrive, without the complications of anxiety and inattention holding him back.)

Attention Development Activities for Infants and Toddlers

It's key to understand that sustained, focused attention is a high-level brain function. This means to excel in this area, kids need a solid foundation of earlier developmental functions to build from. *If* your child is demonstrating any signs of immaturity in the categories of coordination, sensory, and fine motor skills, it will be critical to strengthen those areas of development first. To maximize attentional development, include the exercises and activities in the previous chapters in addition to the strategies shared in this chapter.

Exercise to mature the Moro reflex

- Have your child sit on the edge of a stool or chair. Ask them to cross the right leg over the left leg, and the right arm over the left arm, then curl forward, so their chest is resting on top of their arms and legs and their head is down. Have your child do a big inhale and uncross their arms and legs and extend their arms, legs, and head so the head is tilted back, the arms are fully extended and reaching back, and the legs are spread wide and extended. Then exhale and curl back into the ball position, but change it up, so the left leg is now crossed over the right leg, and the left arm rests on top of the right arm. Repeat ten times while breathing deeply into the belly each time. It's okay to do hand-over-hand guidance to assist your child with the coordination of this exercise. (It's important to note that every child requires a different amount of time to mature the reflex, and it's not unusual for it to take several months to a year to mature beyond this reflex to develop control. Be patient and work this into your daily routine and know that you're also working on coordination and deep breathing, which aid relaxation.)

Activities to engage sustained attention

To exercise and strengthen your child's sustained attention pathways, start with your child's current attentional window of time and slowly increase the amount of time, noting when they begin to wiggle, change the subject, or change tasks. Do a variety of activities, including things they love as well as new, different, and challenging activities that will require effort and practice.

- Read a book
- Sing a song
- Color
- Finger paint
- Build with blocks or Lego® blocks
- Draw a design with sidewalk chalk
- Walk across a balance beam
- Plant seeds in a pot or garden
- Help around the house with a toy broom, vacuum cleaner, lawn mower, or other toys

- Practice counting and recognizing colors and shapes, as well as learning names of body parts, animals, and so on.

Elementary School Students

At this age parents become very aware of their child's attentional abilities through behaviors at home and feedback from teachers. Your child should be having incremental increases in their ability to sit and focus when needed—not just when they choose to sit and focus. Remember that control evolves with development, so kids at this age won't yet have the control of teens or adults to block out distractions and control impulses, but they should demonstrate better control than they had during the preschool years.

Attention Development Milestones for Elementary School Students

Five years:[25]
- Five to ten minutes of sustained attention

Six years:[26]
- Twelve to eighteen minutes of sustained attention

Eight years:[27]
- Sixteen to twenty-four minutes of sustained attention

Ten years:[28]
- Twenty to thirty minutes of sustained attention

Twelve years:[29]
- Twenty-four to thirty-six minutes of sustained attention

The pandemic hit our elementary-aged students hard in terms of school, expectations, and the impact on attention. In many ways, the expectations for our elementary kids during virtual school were the same as for the high school kids: log into Zoom, find and complete assignments online, then submit the assignments virtually. There was no teacher who wandered around the room to ensure you were focused, working, and understanding the assignment. Our elementary kids had all the expectations we had for teenagers but fewer years of development to rise to the challenge.

Add in the impact that stress, change, and the distractions from home had on attention, and the result was a major disruption to attention in our kids for one to two years. On top of that, the increased tech usage meant exercising the reward-driven pathways rather than sustained focused networks.

While we're thrilled to have our kids back in school, we need to step up to support their attention and learning to offset any immaturities and the impact of these past few years. We also need to remember these expectations going forward. While technology can be an asset to teaching and learning, using it with ease and success requires knowledge and experience.

A great starting point for this age, as well as for younger kids, is to use your child's productive window for attention. This helps to set up both you and your child for success, especially when it comes to homework. The challenge is that the amount of homework students are assigned typically has nothing to do with their attentional abilities or age. Your ten-year-old may be on track for their development but if faced with an hour of homework at night is likely to struggle.

I recommend you start with observation at this age as well. That way you can meet your child where they are at this point in terms of attention. Subtly time them while they're doing homework. Start the timer on your phone when they actively engage in their work, not the first time you say, "Time to sit down for spelling practice."

As you're timing, write down notes about how frequently you need to redirect them back to the task and at what point they require redirection after they start their homework. Note when they begin to get fidgety, start to talk off-topic, or make up excuses to take a break. Dropping their pencil, calling the dog over to play, and getting whiny or uncooperative are examples of behaviors you might observe. When you see those actions, you've surpassed their focus window. Also note how fidgety they are when sitting to do work. Is there an occasional swinging of the leg while they're focused, or is it a constant, full-body motion and commotion? This can also provide you with a clue on how to help improve their focus.

What do you do if your child's attentional window is fifteen minutes, but they have an hour's worth of work? Prepare and break it up.

Remember, the brain needs to be rested and fueled to focus. Give the kids a break after school to eat a protein snack—not a snack that's high in sugar—then wait at least twenty minutes for that fuel to kick in. That will help their mood and attitude and ability to focus (see activities list for protein snack ideas). Also, keep in mind that kids have been sitting still and focusing for hours in school all day. Give them a break to move and play before asking them to sit and focus again. This usually helps improve their focus for homework compared to doing it right after school.

Next, create an environment to focus. Do the best you can to remove distractions, which is easier said than done in a household with multiple kids and pets. Think about both visual and noise distractions. Cut out television and music sounds, barking dogs, ringing doorbells, siblings, the ding on your phone from incoming texts—anything you can think of that makes noise.

Think about the best place for the kids to sit to focus. I've always liked my kids to do their homework at the center island in the kitchen. That way I can be unloading the dishwasher or prepping dinner while they're working, and I can help as needed. However, during the pandemic, I learned that they often did better at their desk in the kids' office space we created than in the kitchen. To set up this space we converted the formal living room into their school workspace; it was on the main floor in an open room, where we could keep an eye on things. The kitchen had too many temptations for water and snacks and distractions with two dogs nipping at their feet. Plus, the noises and movement from me making dinner didn't help.

The next key to success is to honor their attention window. This means that when their personal time is up, you either need to let them take a break or step in to provide more help and support, knowing that their focus will be minimal at this point.

If you're anything like me, it's really hard to stop something prior to finishing it. So, if my son's window of focus was up, but he still had two math problems to go, I'd want to push through and have him finish the assignment. If you're going to do that, be prepared for more whining, wiggling, and time to complete the task than if they were fresh and focused.

When deciding whether to push through or take a break, consider a few factors:

- Is it a concept they've already mastered? If they don't understand the concept or haven't memorized the spelling word yet, pushing through will *not* be an effective time to learn.

- How late is it? If taking a break and revisiting the homework will put you past bedtime, staying up even later probably won't help. At that point, it might be best to get the work done and realize that the quality of work and learning will suffer.

- If the studying is important and they still need to learn a concept, the best approach may be to wake up early the next morning to finish studying after a good night's sleep.

- What if your child is a wiggler—that kid who's in constant motion, even when they're focused and working? Excessive fidgeting can be a sign of another possible retained primitive reflex: the spinal galant reflex. This reflex and the Moro reflex are the two reflexes research has shown most commonly linked to ADHD and attentional challenges.[30]

The spinal galant reflex should be present at birth and is not expected to persist beyond twelve months of age. In children who do not integrate this reflex, there can be increased concerns with bladder control, short-term memory issues, difficulty concentrating, and fidgeting.[31] The reflex is activated when there's a stimulus to the back. It causes the hips to move toward the stimulus and is thought to help prepare an infant for crawling. The child who has retained this reflex may move to increase the level of arousal in their brain. It's as though their body craves movement, as the movement sends signals to the brain to increase their level of alertness.

If your child is a wiggler, I recommend doing the spinal galant exercise consistently for several months (see activities section for directions). Even if they've already outgrown this reflex, they'll be engaging in an exercise that provides sensory stimulation to the back and coordinates the limbs. There's no harm in doing this exercise, even if it isn't needed. And if it happens to be needed, you may see less movement and even fewer nighttime accidents, if that's an issue.

I had an interesting conversation about wiggling with Dr. Martin Teicher, a psychiatry professor at Harvard and the director of the Biopsychiatry

Research Program at McLean Hospital. I was spending the day at his lab going through various assessments on myself used for ADHD research, as Dr. Teicher was the lead researcher on a Harvard study of a version of the Brain Balance home program.[32] One of the assessments required staring at a computer screen for twenty minutes and pressing a button when a certain prompt appeared. If you think that sounds awful, you're correct. Twenty minutes feels like hours when doing this task. There are also sensors involved in the task that monitor how much you move during the twenty minutes.

Dr. Teicher shared that while it's known that a child with the hyperactive component of ADHD (ADHD Type 1) will tend to move or wiggle frequently, there can be as much movement involved in the inattentive aspect of ADHD (ADHD Type 2) and ADHD combined (both the hyperactive and inattentive aspects of ADHD). This was new and fascinating to me. We all picture the Type 1 ADHD child as bouncing off the walls, but realizing that inattentive ADHD also involves lots of movement surprised me. He explained that the movements in the inattentive aspect of ADHD are smaller and more subtle. They're movements that would be easy to miss in a classroom, unlike the bigger disruptive movements associated with ADHD Type 1.

Whether the movements distract the child, or the child moves because they're distracted, fidgeting may be a sign of attentional challenges and a need to address the spinal galant reflex.

Another key to attention success is exercise. Dr. John Ratey, author of the book *Spark: The Revolutionary New Science of Exercise and the Brain*, shares a metaphor that "going for a run is like taking a little bit of Prozac and a little bit of Ritalin because, like the drugs, exercise elevates these neurotransmitters."[33] Serotonin, norepinephrine, and dopamine are the neurotransmitters he references because of their influence on attention and learning. Dr. Ratey studied the effects of exercise on cognitive functions, including attention and memory, and found that students performed better following exercise. A key takeaway from his book is that exercise improves learning from several different aspects, including alertness, attention, and motivation.

Exactly how much exercise is needed is still up for debate, and it varies based on your goal. There's benefit in a short burst of activity that spikes the heart rate and engages the muscles, as well as in regularly engaging in sustained activity, such as a thirty-minute run two to three times per week. Tasks that require you to think and coordinate your body have different, but still beneficial, effects on the brain.

There's value in using exercise to prepare to focus as well as to help your child re-engage after taking a break. A homework break doesn't need to be long. In fact, just taking a few minutes to move and engage the muscles can help prepare the brain to be re-engaged to focus. A study out of Western University in London, Canada, found that ten minutes of exercise provided a measurable boost to brain power. Additionally, a meta-review of exercise studies found that short bursts of high-intensity exercises ranging from one to twenty minutes improved brain functions, and the effect lasted up to ten to fifteen minutes.[34] Using exercise as a strategy to prepare to study, as well as taking a short brain break, will help engage additional focus. Exercise has also been shown to enhance memory.[35] The bottom line is you can use exercise before and during homework to help improve productivity.

Attention Development Activities for Elementary School Students

Protein snack ideas to provide a long-lasting fuel to support the brain's ability to focus
- Protein shake, crackers and hummus, toast with peanut butter or other nut butters, banana with peanut butter, oatmeal with a scoop of protein powder or collagen powder, oat balls

Directions for the spinal galant exercise to integrate the reflex
- Have your child lie on their back on a soft surface such as the carpet or a rug. Ask them to slowly move their arms and legs in a snow angel motion, maintaining coordination between the upper and lower body. Move the arms and legs up and out for a three count while doing a deep inhale, then back down for a three count while exhaling. The arms and legs should maintain contact with the ground at all times. If needed to help with coordination of the limbs, you can start with hand-over-hand guidance with your child until they're able to

maintain the pattern on their own. Do a minimum of one set of ten repetitions daily for three to twelve months.

How to plan for homework success

- Work in short chunks of time, based on your child's current attentional window.
- Be sure your child is rested and has had a protein snack twenty minutes prior to focusing.
- Take a break after their window of focus that includes a few minutes of exercise to help re-engage the brain.
- Start with the most difficult tasks that require the most focus.
- If you go beyond their attentional window, be prepared to give more help and guidance—and be prepared for more negative behaviors and less retention of the material.
- Think about where they can do homework that has minimal distractions.
- Exercise to benefit the brain for attention and memory.
- Engage in a sustained exercise activity two to three times a week for thirty minutes.
  - Running, biking, swimming, playing tag, going for a hike, kayaking
- Engage in complex motor activity that requires thought and coordination.
  - Tennis, pickleball, hockey, soccer, football, rock climbing, hopscotch, agility ladder, dance, gymnastics, lacrosse, basketball
- Engage in short but intense bursts of exercise to re-engage focus before and during times when attention is needed.
  - Burpees, jump rope, stair sprints, push-ups, sit-ups, squat jumps—anything to elevate the heart rate
- Refer to the list of activities to engage sustained focus in the toddler section of activities.

Middle School and High School Students

As kids get older, their ability to stay focused for longer increases, but so do the expectations and demands for their attention and organizational abilities. Juggling school, sports, friends, and family can be overwhelming as they learn to navigate life with more independence. **Any attentional difficulties can escalate stress for your child—and family.** Understanding more about attention and ways to improve and maximize these abilities can have an important impact on your child's success and confidence in themselves.

Attention Development Milestones for Middle School and High School Students

If you have a teenager and skipped right to this section, back up. The development of attention, like all aspects of development, involves a sequential chain of events—you can't skip ahead and expect the same level of outcomes.

Fourteen years.[36]
- Twenty-eight to forty-two minutes of sustained attention

Sixteen years.[37]
- Thirty-two to forty-eight minutes of sustained attention

Our middle school and high school kids experienced all the stressors of the younger age groups, but during the pandemic, this age group had the biggest increase in screen time. Technology can have many tremendous benefits, but it can also be a massive drain on our attentional resources, leaving us deficient for other tasks—including the ability to regulate mood and emotions when upset.

A daily structure that balances technology with movement teaches our teens an important strategy for life to support sustained attention, mood, and overall health. We can't expect our kids to choose to put down their devices on their own, so setting expectations and limits to guide them is important at this age. While they can seem so mature in some moments, they're still growing and developing—especially in the regions of the brain responsible for good decision making and impulse control.

Remember Jack, the teen who began failing classes and was having a hard time managing his frustrations and upsets during the pandemic? Jack had a huge lesson on fatigue and the brain one Saturday morning. He was at the halfway point in his program, so I did a few assessment checks with him to monitor his progress. One of the assessments was eye tracking. He did terrible. Far worse than he had done originally—which made no sense at all. He had been working hard and had consistently been improving on his eye coordination and processing exercises. He was so disappointed in his result, and I was confused. I started asking questions about what he had done that morning and the night before. He finally shared that he had stayed up until 3 a.m. gaming. So not only was he tired from lack of sleep, but he had also gamed for over six straight hours. The eye tracking report provided tangible evidence of how prolonged gaming at night crushed attentional and control abilities for the next day. The report showed Jack's eye movements were a mess—on a level you would expect from an elementary-aged child. He had very little control, was overshooting and undershooting the targets, and had slow visual processing and increased errors. In turn, you would then expect his attention and emotional regulation to be on par with a much younger child during that time of brain fatigue as well.

Jack's initial score on the eye tracking assessment was 39/100—low, and with so much room for improvement. His score after the late night of gaming dropped to 17/100.

This is about so much more than just the eyes. Our visual system is highly complex, and analyzing data from eye movements provides indicators to efficacy of attention and control from the brain. This is why eye tracking is used more and more in the concussion world to provide baseline scores for return to play and to illustrate the degree of impact from the concussions.

Discussing Jack's results with him led to a great conversation. I shared with Jack that we measure and analyze eye movements to provide insight into many aspects of brain function, and as we see improvements in eye movements there are also improvements in attention. Through lack of sleep and excessive gaming the night before, Jack lost control of the speed and accuracy of his eye movements. This would also result in a lack of control over other areas as well—his ability to keep his temper in check when frustrated and his ability to focus to do schoolwork. The six hours of gaming crushed his abilities for the next day. Each time he fatigues his brain to this degree, he is going to struggle the next day—with schoolwork, mood, and emotions. He is creating his own uphill battle each time he loses track of time and games for hour after hour.

Jack and I decided to skip his session for that day and instead have him go home and rest. We would try the assessment again one week later—after a good night's sleep and no more than an hour of gaming the night before.

The results of his next eye tracking assessment were a stark contrast from the results after gaming. His eye tracking and processing were much better. The score Jack achieved after rest was 58/100, and assessing this several weeks in a row demonstrated a consistency in this score. While the results still had room for improvement, he had better control, accuracy, speed, and endurance—everything you want in eye movements. He had made great gains compared to his original assessment and night and day results compared to after gaming.

Jack begged me to not show the results to his parents—who were already on him to lessen his gaming. This was physical proof of what they already knew to some degree. I did, of course, show the result to his parents. This was tremendously important information.

While I can't promise that Jack won't continue to have nights he stays up late gaming, I do hope that he thinks about what he needs to do later that day or the next and applies this information to his life and choices.

Not everyone has access to eye tracking technology to observe the impact on their brain and eyes after gaming, but we can communicate this information to our kids and teach them strategies for success and learning to balance the amount of technology usage. Knowing this information doesn't mean they'll always make good life choices—they're still developing teens—but over time and through life lessons, they'll hopefully begin to make the correlation between their actions and their success.

Another critical strategy is for our teens to become aware of what type of attentional systems they're using and how what they do throughout a day impacts their ability to perform.

To have these conversations with your child, start by sharing how you feel and explain what's happening in the brain when you feel that way. Describe how you feel when you're sitting at your computer and staring at the screen but thinking about what you're going to make for dinner. This is an example of using your environmental attention (the default mode network) when you need to be using your focused attention.

If you've just spent a chunk of time scrolling social media, acknowledge that you got sucked into a reward-driven activity where you lose track of time and that you wish you'd done it for less time, since you know that time just burned through energy. Discuss that you just exercised your reward-driven pathways, rather than exercising your sustained attention pathways.

Once you describe how the various types of attention are used and how they impact you, model what you can do to impact your attention in a positive manner. Then share a strategy for each challenge that minimizes your focus.

If your teen is struggling to activate focused attention, have them ask themselves these questions:

1. **Am I rested?** If you're tired, it will be much harder to access your focused attention and to sustain that attention for longer than a few minutes. If you don't have enough time for a good night's sleep or a nap, taking just a few minutes to engage in high-intensity exercise can help to re-ignite your focus for at least a little longer.

2. **Am I hungry?** The brain needs fuel to support the high-level function of sustained attention. Having a healthy snack that includes protein can replenish your reserves to support complex brain activity, including focus.

3. **How stressed am I right now?** I love the quote from Dr. Jha that says, "Stress hijacks your attention."[38] Consider what you can do to reduce your stress. Something as simple as making a to-do list can provide a sense of calm and control.

4. **Am I distracted?** Sensory stimuli can pull your attention and distract you from the task at hand. Minimize sound and visual distractions as much as possible.

5. **Am I trying to juggle too much at once?** Multi-tasking, or task-switching, is one of the fastest ways to burn through your attentional window of opportunity. To help you focus on a single task, turn off the alerts on your phone and computer so you aren't interrupted by texts and emails.

6. **Have I worked too long without taking a break?** We all have a threshold of how long we can maintain our focused attention, and when we go beyond that window we are less effective. Taking a short break to move or eat can help to reset the brain so it is prepared for another window of productive time.

If your kids are anything like mine, they'll roll their eyes when you ask them about these questions or suggest these solutions. But with lots of time and repetition, your voice and message just might stick with them when you're not around to help.

My daughter, Morgan—by accident—shared something with me that showed she just may be listening after all. She always gets extremely nervous before her cross-country races, and after one particular race, she described its debacle.

Morgan started the race strong and was in second place behind her good friend. We saw all the girls run into the woods, then we saw girl after girl run out—but no Morgan. Eventually she emerged, running hard and looking strong.

"What the heck? Did she stop and walk?" my husband asked.

After Morgan cooled down, we went to check on her and find out what happened.

She said, "You know how you always say stress makes it hard for your brain to work? That's what happened! I was so stressed I couldn't think at all!"

She explained how she made a wrong turn on the cross-country course and led an entire section of girls down the wrong path. She'd been in second place, but her teammate was far enough ahead that she couldn't see where she was. And then she turned too soon and followed a path that eventually came to a dead end. When she saw the dead end, she turned around and told the girls behind her they'd gone the wrong way. They all turned around and headed back out, with Morgan trailing in the back of the pack.

The team had walked the course before the race, but because she was so stressed, she struggled to pay attention and then couldn't remember the course. Luckily, Morgan could laugh at herself over the mishap, and she learned the hard way how important it is to pay close attention to the pre-race walk-through—especially when she's stressed.

In addition to building awareness about attention and how it can be minimized, it's also important to strengthen focused attention through practice. At this age more than the others, kids need to spend time using both environmental attention and sustained, focused attention. They get plenty of time strengthening their reward-driven attention through gaming, texting, and social media. We need to help them strengthen the other aspects of attention so they have balanced abilities.

While it may sound funny to practice using your environmental focus, it's becoming more and more necessary to be intentional about this time. Notice how often you spend time *not* actively engaged in something—it's more rare than you think! For me, that's when I'm showering and getting ready for the day, driving in the car by myself, or going for a run. But even that time can be disrupted if you're not careful. Listening to a podcast instead of music while running or getting ready for the day turns your free time for roaming thoughts, creativity, and processing emotions into actively engaged time. When you're driving in your car and reach for your phone at a stoplight, you're once again interrupting the free time you have, distracting yourself from your own thoughts. Instead, you're aimlessly scrolling social media or reading a text.

Your environmental focus time is when you process your life, review your past, plan for the future, and brainstorm. Your thoughts will naturally bounce from topic to topic. This isn't ADHD unless it is interfering with life, learning, and interactions. A mind that wanders when not engaged in a specific task is appropriate; this is normal and good. This is your time to daydream, to have introspection and understand what's happening in your life and how it makes you feel. This time also contributes to memory retrieval.[39] Our kids *need* this time to absorb what's happening in life and to face their own thoughts and feelings. This kind of focus (or non-focus) burns a low amount of fuel but continues to engage and strengthen an aspect of attention. I always think of this time as "free-range thinking" and try to ensure I carve out time each day to exercise these pathways to process life and create space for creativity.

If you create times when everyone sets aside their phones to just *be*, you'll be providing time for environmental focus. Create a routine where no one's on their phone in the car and you have that time of silence, or only have the radio playing in the background, so you have time to daydream. Encourage your kids to exercise with music, not podcasts. Take time to relax by taking a long bath or just going for a walk. Create opportunities to build habits that include downtime and time for free-range thinking.

Sometimes our own thoughts can be uncomfortable and even stressful. This can contribute to us doing things to avoid facing our thoughts, fears, and worries. Watching a show, scrolling the internet, reading a book, and using drugs and alcohol are all examples of ways that we can shut off our thoughts. It's important for our kids to learn to be with their thoughts, especially during times of stress. Not only will this contribute to processing their experiences and emotions, but it will also help them practice pushing through tough times.

While it's beneficial to have time when you're not engaged in anything specific, it's also beneficial to intentionally engage in meditation. Learning to meditate and creating a habit of meditating regularly may be one of the best tactics to improve focus and help manage stress. In one study, mindfulness meditation was found to improve one's attention in a way that allows a person to block out distractions and focus on a single task.[40] Wikipedia describes mindfulness as, "The practice of purposely bringing one's attention to the present-moment experience without evaluation, a skill one develops through meditation or other training."[41] While it's not fully understood how mindfulness meditation improves attention, there are now hundreds of studies dedicated to deepening this understanding.[42] Meditation has been shown to decrease activation in the part of your brain involved in your fight or flight response, the part that's activated during times of extreme stress, fear, or anger. It also increases activation in higher-functioning regions of the brain that contribute to sustained attention, impulse control, and decision making.[43] According to the *Harvard Business Review*, spending just ten to fifteen minutes a day meditating changes the way we engage with ourselves, others, and our work.[44]

Attention Development Activities for
Middle School and High School Students

See previous sections on activities for toddlers and elementary school kids for additional categories and ideas to support strengthening sustained attention.

- Build self-awareness of your current attentional state.
  - As parents, comment on what you notice about your own attention and what you can do to improve it.
  - Ask questions about what your child notices in themselves—when their attention is going well and when it isn't.
- Work with your child to create a to-do list, and next to each item mark the type of attention needed to accomplish the task. Then help them plan their day so that the tasks that require focused attention are done at a time they will be alert and fed, not tired and hungry. Provide breaks for movement if there are multiple items on the list that require sustained focus. Examples of possible tasks and the type of attention they require are:
  - Going for a run—environmental focus
  - Reading a chapter in a novel for school they enjoy—sustained attention (but since it is a book they like, it will require less effort and resources than reading something highly complex)
  - Studying for a chemistry text—sustained attention (with high levels of fuel demands because difficult)
  - Math homework—sustained attention (recommend to do an exercise or movement break between studying for chemistry and math to re-engage attention and focus)
  - Unloading the dishwasher—environmental focus
- Create time and space for your kids for "free-range thinking," time to simply be with their thoughts, not actively engaged in any other tasks.
- Exercise. Different types of exercise support attention and learning in different ways, so it's good to engage in a variety of exercise.
  - High-intensity bursts of exercise
  - Sustained exercise

- º Complex motor movements
- Practice mindfulness meditation.
  - º Just ten minutes a day can improve focus, awareness of self, memory, and more.
  - º Many free or inexpensive apps exist for mindfulness meditation
- Use time blocking.
  - º During busy times of juggling school and life, work with your teen using a daily planner to map out time blocking. Set designated times to get work done and set all other things aside (phone, email, etc.).
- Plan tech usage.
  - º Use tech after homework is completed, on the weekend—times when decreased focus and regulation after usage won't negatively impact school or family interactions.
- To build awareness and understanding around the impact of tech usage, track usage and rate mood, energy, and focus after usage—thirty minutes, one hour, two hours. Mood and habit tracking apps such as Daylio and Moodfit track lifestyle elements, including sleep and exercise, to help build awareness around the impact of life on mood!

Signs That Indicate Improvement

Improvements in your child's attention and focus will be subtle but noticeable if you are observant. Over time you'll notice your child staying engaged in homework for longer periods of time and acting more independently and with fewer reminders to stay focused. As focus increases, you'll also note improvements in impulse control and organization—your child will have a better ability to plan and manage time and prioritize. Confidence in self and abilities, consistent work and follow-through, and better attention to details are other bonuses that can go along with improved attention. As their attentional awareness and abilities strengthen over time you will notice an improvement in their time management and maximizing their day for productivity. Improving their ability to manage time and accomplish tasks feels good and can contribute to their sense of self and ability to tackle hard things and succeed.

5

. . . .

RELATIONSHIPS— DEVELOPING SOCIAL AND COMMUNICATION SKILLS

The year 2020 came with many experiences and life lessons. For me, one of the strongest messages was a reminder about the importance of human connection—and it became evident through the *absence* of it. Before this time, we took so much for granted: spending time with family, friends, and neighbors; impromptu driveway gatherings on a gorgeous evening; planned dinners out with friends; time with extended family. Those face-to-face interactions when we laughed, shared, and caught up on life deepened our connections and relationships and gave us a sense of community, belonging, and fulfillment. When all that was stripped away, many people felt more isolated and alone in a time of exaggerated stress. Eventually the social distancing and masks became less common, then went away, but our lives experienced so many changes that not everything returned to the way it once was. These changes especially impacted friendships and connections in adolescent children during a time in their lives when their sense of belonging is largely impacted by their peers and friendships. Adolescents, more than other age groups, experienced loneliness during the pandemic, with a 2021 study reporting twice as many teens struggling with feelings of loneliness compared to ten years ago.[1] Not only were they cut off from peers, they were also cut off from important development opportunities, and the impact has become clear.

Note to Parents

Social development begins in infancy with the bonding between parent and child and continues to expand beyond parents over time. Social interactions begin with observation and awareness and evolve into play and interactions, and these relationships provide learning, fulfillment, and often joy. Making the time to prioritize connection and interaction is key for *all* ages—kids and adults. Supporting the development and well-being of our kids also means that we as parents foster and support deep and meaningful friendships and relationships for ourselves. As adults, juggling all that goes into family and schedules at this stage of life, it is too easy to set aside our own needs. Be intentional about nurturing meaningful friendships for yourself as well as for your kids. Not only will this model a healthy variety of relationships but it can also contribute to creating your community of love and support.

While the social needs for teens are widely known, they weren't the only age group to experience a developmental impact from the reduction in socialization. "Children are not getting the cognitive and social stimulation that they would normally get outside their home," said Dr. Michelle Aguilar, the head of pediatrics at Venice Family Clinic in Los Angeles, California. "Providers have noted delays in speech and language as well as trouble sharing and being in groups."[2]

While life after the pandemic slowly shifted back to a more familiar landscape, it isn't as simple as picking up where we left off. Time passed, which created gaps in both the underlying development of our youth and the learning curve that comes with practice on top of that neurological development. We need to learn from this time and apply these reminders to support our kids going forward—creating time and opportunities for them to build meaningful connections and relationships with their peers.

The ability to interact in an age-appropriate manner with peers, to communicate, to listen, and to engage, can't develop unless the brain accurately perceives and interprets social cues and information. Further, social learning involves practice—our social skills improve over years through trial and error. When a child is playing on the playground and yells at a friend, then that friend leaves, they learn the lesson that, "When I yell at my friend, they leave. If I want to keep playing with my friend, I need to handle that differently." The temporary pause on group sports and activities, school playground and cafeteria time, and playdates stopped the learning curve that comes with peer interactions.

Pandemic Lessons

The change and reduction in social interactions were stark reminders on many levels of the importance of human connection, friendships, and relationships. The isolation, loneliness, and depression that resulted across the age-span during the pandemic lockdown illustrated this impact. There were also those who for many reasons thrived during the pandemic. There was a relief in slowing the pace of life, and for kids who were experiencing bullying or difficult peer interactions, this pause provided a reprieve. While this break was beneficial to some, it wasn't an ideal environment to continue to foster social/emotional development in our kids. Interacting with parents and siblings is not the same as learning from nuanced interactions with friends and classmates.

The impact varied by age. The scientific journal *Nature* published a study that found that during the pandemic, six-month-old infants were assessed as being behind in communication.[3] Toddlers had fewer opportunities to observe other kids and to learn to share and to play through interactions with peers. Our elementary-aged kids lost time on the playground, where they would have learned to navigate hurt feelings, upsets, and celebrations with friends. Middle school kids, who crave belonging, were left to struggle to fit in and connect through texts, FaceTime, and social media. Communicating behind the veil of technology, they were unable to interpret tone, sarcasm, and the nuances of communication that give meaning to our interactions. Often, their social engagement came through Snapchat photos and texts, receiving likes on a post, or, adversely, observing when friends got together without them.

While we can't undo the past, we can learn from the impact and create space to build friendships and relationships, to set aside technology and interact face to face, to practice communication and empathy, and to find joy collectively.

Science Alert

A Harvard study that examined relationships over seventy-five years found that the emotional, physical, and mental quality of our lives is directly proportional to the quality of our relationships.[4] But building relationships takes time, intentional effort, and communication.

Adults have spent decades communicating, and we may take for granted the numerous skills that coalesce to be an effective communicator, such as the ability to listen, to not only hear but also process what the other person says. We've learned how to interpret the nuances of body language and tone of voice. We've had lots of practice recognizing our feelings and emotions and putting them into words, then sharing those words with someone else. Not only do those aspects of communication require practice, but many brain networks and regions are involved that must work together in perfect harmony. Communication and socialization are dependent on the brain and its development of the many pathways working together.

Infants and Toddlers

Infants' social interactions begin with making simple eye contact, watching facial expressions, and listening to tone of voice. Over time these interactions transition to conversational babble, then actions and noises to capture and hold the attention of caregivers and to communicate needs. Playing peekaboo and repeatedly dropping a toy so that it is picked back up again are both examples of early socialization. This involves trial and error and repeating the same actions over and over to learn what to expect. Building a social foundation as an infant or toddler engages curiosity—they need to watch and learn from the people in their lives.

Relationship and Social Development
Milestones for Infants and Toddlers

Socialization and communication milestones[5]
Two months:

- Looks at your face, smiles when you talk to them

Four months:

- Smiles or makes noises to get or hold your attention; makes cooing sounds such as *oohhh, ahhh*; makes sounds back when you talk to them

Six months:

- Knows familiar people, likes to look at self in the mirror, laughs, takes turns making sounds with you, blows raspberries (sticks tongue out and blows), makes squealing noises

Nine months:

- Acts shy, clingy, or fearful around strangers; shows several facial expressions—happy, sad, angry, surprised; reacts when you leave (looks, cries, or reaches for you); reacts with smiles or laughs when playing peekaboo; lifts arms to be picked up; makes babbling noises with consonant sounds: *dadadada, mamama, babababa*

Twelve months:

- Plays games with you such as pat-a-cake, waves bye-bye, calls parent *mama/dada*, understands *no* and will briefly pause when you say it

Fifteen months:

- Copies other children when playing; takes a toy out of a container when another child does it; shows you objects they like; claps when excited; hugs stuffed dolls or toys; shows you affection with hugs, kisses, and cuddles; tries to say one or two words besides *mama/dada* (*ba* for ball, *da* for dog); looks at a familiar object when you name it (*ball, dog*); follows directions if you prompt with word and gesture (holding out your hand and saying, "give me the toy"); points to something to show you what they want

Eighteen months:

- Moves away from you but will look to be sure you are close by; points to show you something interesting; helps you dress them by working with you (pushes arm through sleeve or lifts up foot for pants); tries to say three or more words; follows one-step directions without gestures

Two years:

- Notices when others are hurt or upset; will pause or look sad when someone is crying; looks at your face to see how to react in a new situation; points to things in a book when you ask, "Where is the bear?"; says at least two words together, like "more milk"; uses more gestures than just waving and pointing, like blowing kisses or nodding head *yes*

Two to three years:[6]

- Asks for wants; has little interaction with other kids (engages in more parallel play with peers than interactive or collaborative play—they are interested in observing other kids, but play remains focused on themselves); expresses affection warmly; develops rituals and routines

Thirty months:

- Plays next to other children and sometimes plays with them; shows you what they can do; says "Look at me!"; follows simple routines when told, like helping to pick up toys when you say, "It's cleanup time"; says about fifty words; says two or more together with one action word, for example, "doggie run"; names things in a book when you point and ask "What is this?"; says words like *I*, *me*, or *we*

Three years:

- Calms down within ten minutes after you leave them at childcare; notices other children and joins them to play; talks with you in a conversation using at least two back-and-forth exchanges; asks, "who, what, where, or why" questions, like "Where is Mommy/Daddy?"; says what action, like running, eating, or playing, is happening in a picture when asked; says first name when asked; talks well enough for others to understand most of the time

Four years:

- Pretends to be something else (teacher, superhero, dog) during play; asks to play with other children if none are around; comforts others who are hurt or sad, for example, hugs a crying friend; likes to be a helper; changes behavior based on place (place of worship, library, playground); says sentences with four or more words; says some words from a song, story, or nursery rhyme; talks about at least one thing that happened during the day: "I played soccer"; answers simple questions: "What is a coat for?" or "What is a crayon for?"

The simplest place to start for social development in young kids is with exposure to people. And not just people, but people who aren't wearing masks. Every person has a rich array of both facial features and expressions. Being able to recognize and identify emotions and expressions takes repetition and practice—seeing what *happy* looks like on your face, then seeing what *happy* looks like on their grandmother, their neighbor, the postal worker, your friends, your friends' kids, the grocery store checkout person, and so on. While there are consistencies regarding what *happy* looks like, each person's anatomy and expression will be uniquely their own. It's important to find a way to provide these experiences for your child.

During the pandemic, infants and toddlers experienced less variety in interactions with others and sometimes had less face-to-face interaction with those they saw daily. Siblings and parents worked and schooled from home, and they were often absorbed in technology. Our little ones thrive on direct attention. By setting aside work or technology for just a few minutes, you can engage face to face and provide meaningful interactions.

Being exposed to different faces, expressions, and interactions will not only begin to build your child's catalogue of awareness, it will also exercise their abilities to interact. Remember that babies as young as four months will make noises to try to capture and hold your attention; they are aware of your interactions and are demanding them in their own way. Babies at six months begin to engage in back-and-forth "conversation" with their coos and babbling sounds.

I learned this as a young child from my little sister. I'm nine years older than my youngest sister, Lisa. When she was an infant, I read parts of a parenting book my mom had sitting out (because what nine-year-old wouldn't read a book about development—clearly I was interested in this topic decades before I realized it). While I don't remember the name of the book, I do remember the gist of what it taught me. The book talked about the importance of mimicking a baby's babble. This was hilarious to me, and I decided to give it a try. I'd lie on the floor with baby Lisa and imitate every little noise and coo she made. She loved this and would play along nicely, kicking, squealing, and cooing away. We'd go back and forth, and it entertained us both for quite some time. Then, I noticed something. Not only would Lisa go back and forth with me and take turns, she also tried to copy what I was doing with my face and sometimes even my sounds. If I did a surprised face, with my mouth in the shape of an *o,* she did the same with her mouth. She watched me intently, then did her best to imitate what she saw.

Years later, I remembered this and did the same thing with my own babies. I held them on my lap with our faces just inches apart and made faces and noises back and forth with them. I found that same connection, interaction, and mimicking. All that silliness was laying the groundwork for those beginning pieces of communication and socializing.

Another fundamental aspect of social interaction is verbal communication, which includes both the words themselves and our ability to organize those words into sentences and expressions that others can understand and follow. Verbal communication doesn't begin with actual words but with a chain of developmental steps that gives a baby the ability to control the movement of their mouth in order to generate sounds and eventually words. A key primitive reflex, the rooting reflex, helps from day one to drive this progression of development.

The rooting reflex is a reflex that you're most likely familiar with. When you touch the corner of an infant's mouth, or even their cheek, they turn their head in the hopes of eating. Touching their cheek provides sensory input to their face, bringing awareness to the brain of that sensation. The brain responds to that sensory input by activating muscles to turn the head toward the stimulation and thrust the tongue forward. When there's light stimulation to the roof of the baby's mouth, it triggers the sucking and swallowing reflex, activating additional muscle movements and the epiglottis—the flap in the throat that closes off while eating, so food and liquids don't enter the lungs.[7] This practice begins to build the neural connections to perceive sensation and to control muscles and movement.

We have a great picture of Morgan as a brand-new baby, firmly latched on to Doug's T-shirt as Doug is laughing and saying, "Wrong parent, little one!" The instinct is strong, and it engages the muscles in the mouth, which over time develop the strength and coordination to move solid food around in the mouth, to chew and swallow, and to enunciate words.

Similar to other primitive reflexes we've discussed, an infant will outgrow the rooting reflex by four to six months of age, when their brain learns to override the reflex and develop conscious control over the reaction to facial touch stimuli and mouth movements.[8] **However, if a child is delayed in outgrowing the rooting reflex, there can be a higher incidence of motor and speech delays and other complications.**

Travis was a preschooler who'd been working with a speech therapist prior to the pandemic. He had great receptive language—meaning that he understood what his parents were saying to him—but he was behind in his speech and enunciation. He knew what he wanted, but often his parents and siblings couldn't figure out what he was trying to communicate, which resulted in tears and meltdowns.

When the pandemic hit and speech shifted to Zoom sessions with his therapist, his mom felt stuck. It was hard for the therapist to hold Travis's attention at such a young age through the computer, and his mom felt the sessions weren't productive. She ended up halting those sessions but didn't want to wait until the pandemic was over to help Travis. She called me to ask if I had any suggestions.

I told her that I wasn't sure if I'd have helpful recommendations but would know more if I could meet Travis. We set up another Zoom call, and I promised I'd only need about five minutes with him. I talked her through stroking his cheek from the corner of his mouth outward lightly, so I could check his rooting reflex. Sure enough, even though Travis was four, there was a slight but quick cheek twitch each time she stroked his cheek. He had this reaction on both sides, but it was much stronger on the right. Travis still retained the rooting reflex. We checked a few of his other reflexes, too, and found that several were still present. While I'm never happy to see a child with reflexes still present, it always gives me hope because I know there's room for improvement, and there's a scientific reason for the complications. This isn't a lazy kid who wants to point to objects rather than use words. This is a kid who has a reduced ability to coordinate the muscles of his mouth and tongue to form and coordinate the movements for speech.

I taught Travis and his mom how to do the exercises for the rooting reflex, as well as the other exercises for his retained primitive reflexes. I also recommended that even though Travis was four, his mom should play the mirror game each day with facial expressions and make it a silly, fun, and playful time. His mom would mirror his funny face and make him guess her emotion or what made her happy/scared/tired. She used that time to connect face to face, to laugh, snuggle, and engage while building Travis's brain and body to better prepare him for speech and communication.

When Travis's speech therapist reached back out for in-person sessions, she was shocked. Travis had grown by leaps and bounds during his break and had closed a large portion of his language gap. They picked up not where they left off but much further down the list of their goals. The rooting reflex exercise was not a replacement for his speech therapy, but maturing this aspect of development helped to contribute to the work he was doing to enhance his speech.

As a parent, it can be hard to know whether your child is right on track or has an area of need. We all watch, worry, and analyze. We all fill out the checklists at the pediatrician's office, but there's so much more to your child than what a checklist and a short appointment can determine. Spending time with playgroups and with other parents and kids of similar ages can be a powerful support element for fostering relationships and growth in both kids and parents.

The need for group time and interactions struck me early in my years at Brain Balance. I noticed a trend: if a child was an oldest child, or an only child, the parent often came in with less understanding or awareness of their child's struggle and their degree of difficulty. These parents usually wanted to know if what they were experiencing was normal or if they should worry.

"He's fine. He's just a bit of a handful when he's upset," they'd say.

Then I'd hear parents describe a typical example of the child's behavior and would think, "Holy cow! Not only is that stressful, but that is *not* what a typical meltdown or tantrum looks like for a four-year-old!"

In contrast, conversations with parents who had multiple kids often started further down the path. These parents already knew something was amiss or different with their child. They'd already accepted that, and they were looking for guidance to create change.

There's value in spending lots of time with kids who are similar in age to your own and their parents. Observing your child while they play alongside others can help you see not only differences in personalities but also if the elements of development are veering off track. If you notice something's awry, trust your gut. No one knows your child the way you do. But rest assured, you don't need to lose sleep or panic; it's simply information. Now you have an opportunity to support your child going forward.

Relationship and Social Development
Activities for Infants and Toddlers

- The rooting reflex: Engage the rooting reflex through sensory stimulation on the face. Touch, tickle, rub, kiss your baby's cheeks. Stimulate the face from the corners of the mouth out toward the ears. For older kids you can use your finger to draw imaginary lines on the cheeks going from the cheek in toward the mouth, or from the corner of the mouth outward. Be sure to engage both sides. Continue to engage and stimulate until your child no longer turns toward the sensation. The amount of time needed varies but can take daily engagement for three to twelve months. You should no longer see any twitching or reacting from the mouth or a need to "wipe away" the sensory stimulus by using their hand to rub where they felt the sensation.

- Mimic sounds and babble to engage in "conversation," going back and forth with your baby.

- Make an exaggerated facial expression for your baby to imitate—happy, sad, surprised—and, as they get older, name the expression. Have your child call out an expression you have to act out. Mimic their face and guess their expression. Play games and talk about what made you happy, sad, angry, or scared (can be real or make-believe). When you act out an expression, point out aspects of your body language: "When I am sad, my face is sad, and my body may look sad with a droopy expression and droopy shoulders."

- Play pretend. Pick up a pencil and say, "Meet Bobby. Bobby is a rabbit who likes to hop . . ." and tell a made-up story. If your child is older, ask them to participate. "What do you think Bobby should do next? Should he hop on your head? Should he hop over to say hi to our dog?"

- Create a weekly playgroup with kids similar in age, meet weekly with a group at a local park or nature center, go to the library for story time, find a moms' group online or through a religious body or pediatrician's office, or start a meet-up group.
- Have your baby play in front of a mirror. Put a hat on their head or a sticker on their nose, play peekaboo. Notice when your baby realizes that the baby in the mirror is themselves.
- Optimize opportunities for your baby to see many different people. Go to the grocery store, coffee shop, department store, and local farmer's market on the weekend. Watch a kids' soccer game, even if you don't know anyone. There will be dozens of kids and families running around. In the summer, go to an outdoor family concert or music/theater in the park.
- Play with bubbles, using the wand and blowing.
- Blow air through a straw, aiming at a target. Blow the straw wrapper across the table at a restaurant.

Elementary School Students

Kids at this age will develop friendships with a "bestie"—one close friend—and a wider group of friends that may shift throughout the school year. They can be very sensitive to feeling left out and develop a heightened sense of awareness of what is fair, right, and wrong in play and games. It's a fun time of exploring and developing a wider range of interests and activities. As their self-awareness increases, they can begin to be more critical of themselves and their abilities. In addition to the academic learning that happens at this age, this is also a time of powerful social/emotional learning, which is just as critical to their overall well-being. They are beginning to be more aware of others and how their actions impact others. The development of empathy and reading nonverbal social cues is happening through trial, error, and repetition at this age as well.

Relationship and Social Development Milestones
for Elementary School Students

Five years:[9]

- Tells a story they heard or made up with at least two events (for example, a cat was stuck in a tree and a firefighter saved it)
- Answers simple questions about a book or story after you read or tell it to them
- Keeps a conversation going with more than three back-and-forth exchanges
- Uses or recognizes simple rhymes, for example, *bat/cat, ball/tall*
- Follows rules or takes turns when playing games with other children
- Sings, dances, or acts for you
- Does simple chores at home like matching socks or clearing the table after eating
- Knows words are made of different sounds and syllables
- Can identify words with the same beginning sound (example: *mommy* and *marshmallow*)
- Can use correct form of verbs to talk about past and future events[10]

Five to six years:[11]

- Speech should be grammatically correct, on the whole (correct most of the time based on what has been modeled at home)
- Questions things more deeply, addressing meaning and purpose
- Changes friendships rapidly
- Leads as well as follows
- Chooses own friends
- Engages other children in play or role assignments
- Apologizes for mistakes
- Begins to learn sounds that go with letters of the alphabet
- Learns that individual sounds combine together to form words
- Starts to understand that single words may have multiple meanings and begins to use context to know what the word means

- Understands they can make new words by joining two other words (*dog/house*)
- Learns that the beginnings and endings of words can change their meanings (*happy/happiness, teach/teacher*)

Six years:[12]

- Begins to read simple stories of words that are spelled the way they sound (example: *pig*)

Six to seven years:[13]

- Has ability to describe experiences
- Talks about thoughts and feelings
- Masters pronunciation of consonants *f, v*
- Pronounces *sh, ch, th*
- Can tell a complicated story
- Wants to be the first and best at everything
- Focuses less on self and shows more concern for others
- Develops a positive, realistic self-concept
- Gains awareness of own feelings
- Begins to learn from mistakes
- May become infatuated with teacher or playmate
- Can be jealous of others and siblings[14]

Seven to eight years:[15]

- Cares for self, room, and belongings
- Has a sense of humor and tells jokes
- Draws moral distinctions based on internal judgment
- Is self-critical
- May express lack of confidence
- Dislikes being singled out, even for praise
- Develops a sense of responsibility

Eight years:[16]

- Can write a simple story

Eight to nine years:[17]

- Can converse at an almost adult level
- Able to write simple compositions

- Becomes impatient
- Finds waiting for special events torturous
- Is influenced by peer pressure
- Seeks immediate gratification
- Actively seeks out praise
- Fears speaking in front of class
- Is self-critical
- Is highly social

Nine to ten years:[18]

- Can express a wide range of emotions
- Is both industrious and impatient
- Wants to put some distance between self and adults
- Understands roles and appropriate behavior and considers them inflexible
- Can be aloof
- Has more stable emotions than in previous years
- Controls anger

Ten to eleven years:[19]

- Shows interest in teen culture (music, social media, makeup)
- Tries to avoid looking childish
- Understands how behavior affects others
- Is truthful
- Is proud of doing things well
- Succumbs to peer pressure more readily
- Is increasingly self-conscious
- Enjoys using the phone[20]
- Friends are important and may have a best friend

Eleven to twelve years:[21]

- May be a repeat of the terrible twos
- Tries to establish independence and autonomy
- Tends to gossip and talk about others
- Can adapt behavior to fit situation
- Exhibits off-color humor and silliness

- Has little impulse control
- Enjoys recreational activities
- Is energetic and enthusiastic
- Is easily frustrated
- May feel out of control

As you continue to support your child's social and emotional development, know that the elements of development can move at different paces. This means your child can be brilliant and ahead of their peers in one area but still behind in another area. Celebrating their strengths and acknowledging and supporting their growth opportunities will better prepare them to interact with their peers and build meaningful relationships.

All too often I hear parents share a concern and then minimize or discredit it. Having an area of strength does not negate an area of challenge.

"He's a really social kid. He *wants* friends but doesn't always know when to back off. But he's so smart, above and beyond his peers when it comes to math, so I know he'll be okay."

Being smart and being socially aware and appropriate are two different areas of the brain that don't cancel each other out. It's not unusual for a child to excel in one area and struggle in another, and the good news is, it's possible to improve the areas of challenge to minimize the struggle. A strength does not cancel out a weakness. Both can and do exist at the same time and will complicate life.

Social immaturity can be harder to discern, especially in younger years when birthday party invitations are extended to the entire class. It's easy to mistake frequent party invitations as a sign that the child has a lot of friends. You'll need to look beyond the party invitations to be confident that your child is on track in terms of social development and engagement.

Watch your child's interactions in a large group of kids with varying ages. Kids (and adults) naturally gravitate to those with similar interests and levels of development. If your child tends to play with kids a few years younger—or even several years older—this can be a red flag and you should watch closely. Kids who struggle to read nonverbal social cues or to interact with their same-aged peers are often more accepted by younger kids, who are at that same level, and older kids who have more patience and awareness.

Another red flag is when your child is frequently upset while playing with others. If he or she often comes home with hurt feelings or distressed, this is a good reason to spend some time observing them at play. There are times when the upset is warranted, but there are also times when a child misinterprets the scenario and gets their feelings hurt. The younger a child is, the more frequent and dramatic the upsets. If this feels like a description of your child, know that their behavior is providing you a clue to an area of immature development—an immaturity in social interactions, control and/or inhibition that is a result of development.

My sister Lisa (whom I told you about) had this experience of a misinterpretation when she was a coach at Brain Balance. Lisa had been an elementary school teacher for several years prior to joining the Brain Balance team. She was firm and had high expectations for the kids but celebrated their wins every step of the way, and the kids loved working with her. Except for one fifth-grade student, named Alex. His mom came to me one day asking if he could change coaches. She said that Alex felt like coach Lisa didn't like him, and it made him uncomfortable. I agreed with the mom that working with someone you thought didn't like you wouldn't be fun. I let her know that prior to changing his coach, I wanted to dig in a little further, since this did not sound like Lisa at all. I spoke with Alex before the session, and he said that most of the time with Lisa it was fun, but when they shifted to book work, he felt like she got mad at him. I told Alex that I would observe his session, and whenever he felt uncomfortable, he should use a code word, *nachos,* so I'd know how he felt.

Alex and Lisa made it about forty-five minutes before I heard the word *nachos* during the reading section. I had them pause the session and took Alex aside to thank him for using the code word and ask what prompted him to use it. He said Lisa looked angry, but he didn't know why. Knowing my sister well, I assured him that was definitely not her angry face. I asked Alex to sit with me to observe Lisa reading with the next student, so he could show me when she made that face again.

"Nachos!" he said again. When I looked at her face, it all clicked into place. Lisa had her "thinking" face on as she corrected the work, read through the answers, and wrote out the feedback. She was deep in thought. Her brow was furrowed as she was deeply engaged with what she was reading and correcting.

Then Lisa, Alex, and I sat down together to do a little role play. I asked Lisa to show us her happy face, then her mad face, and finally her thinking face. When Alex saw her actual mad face, he could see the difference between her mad and thinking face, and he realized she hadn't been mad at him after all. Lisa's stern/mad teacher face was eyes wide, brows up, and head back in a "you've got to be kidding me" type expression, versus the furrowed brow of concentration.

We made a game of this scenario going forward. We gave Alex a buzzer, and every time Lisa had her thinking face on, he hit the buzzer, which brought awareness to them both and turned it into a fun game—but one where learning was still happening for Alex.

While a fifth grader may seem too old to play a facial expression game, it was what he needed. When a child is unsure of how to interpret something, it's easy to take things personally. This can result in hurt feelings and upsets that aren't necessary. This is also a red flag of developmental immaturity in the child's ability to feel and process their own body, making it hard for them to be aware of their own nonverbal social cues. This lack of awareness of self makes it harder to interpret this information in someone else.

After you've observed your child's social interactions and have a better sense of their developmental abilities with communication, socialization, and behaviors, then it's time to adjust your expectations. This doesn't mean you let them get away with things; this means you're going to set expectations based on their actual abilities, not how you wish they were functioning.

You wouldn't put a three-year-old in kindergarten and expect them to do well. They would require constant redirection to listen, sit back down, and keep their hands to themselves. While they'd learn a few new words, they'd struggle to keep up with all the material. A three-year-old would interact and play with the other kids differently than the five- and six-year-olds.

While this example may sound silly, it's like the expectations we put on our kids. We tend to set expectations based on their age rather than their abilities. How many times have you said, "You're ten, you should be able to look people in the eyes when talking to them/not interrupt a conversation/ not call names when mad/hang up your wet towel/brush your teeth without a dozen reminders."

When we set expectations based on age, we may be setting our kids up to fail. Instead, be realistic about what they can do—how they interact with peers, handle frustrations and upsets—and set your expectations at that level. Then actively work with your child to enhance their development, and, as they mature, you can raise your expectations as their abilities grow.

If your child is seven but gravitates toward younger kids in the neighborhood, isn't riding a bike, and struggles to explain how they feel and why they're upset, their development may be behind. Even though they're in second grade, aspects of their development may be more like those of a kindergartner. To set expectations and support your child, think about what you would expect from a kindergartner.

While with friends, a kindergartner would need occasional reminders to take turns letting other kids be the leader or call the shots. There could be tears when frustrations or upsets happen, and they may not be able to explain why. They may choose to play with different kids each day and may not have one best friend. Their interests and play may gravitate toward make-believe—playing a superhero, teacher, or firefighter.

Think about how you would prepare a five-year-old for an event. You'd talk them through what to expect and prompt or redirect them to use kind words, remember their manners, or apologize when needed.

If you expect seven-year-old behaviors but their development is not ready to support that, you're asking more than what they can do at this time. It will be exhausting for both of you.

Interpreting body language and expression is another key aspect to developing social interactions and communication. But before your child can do this, they must first have an awareness of their own body posture, gestures, and nuances and know how that relates to their moods and emotions. **To identify a mood or emotion in someone else, you first need to be aware** of it in yourself. Sensory perception—including proprioception, your awareness of your body in space—is a foundational element to social communication. (Which is why you shouldn't skip any chapters in this book. Development is all interrelated and builds on itself.)

I can recognize confusion in someone else because I know that when I'm confused, I furrow my brow, tilt my head to the side, and squint my eyes as I ponder what I'm trying to comprehend. If I was unable to sense my body posture and position or couldn't identify my feeling, it would make it much more difficult to identify frustration in someone else. Teachers say this in the classroom all the time: "I see lots of confusion on your faces right now, so let's back up and explain this math problem again." They're bringing awareness to how the kids look and feel. We can apply that same concept with our kids.

One of the best ways to drive awareness about social interactions is to improve a child's proprioception, and when this kicks in for a child, it can be one of the most rewarding aspects of enhancing their development. It helps them fit in, so they can not only make but keep good friends.

Daniel was a great example of this. He was the oldest in a family of five kids in a neighborhood filled with kids. Even during the pandemic, the kids continued to play together outside. The doorbell rang constantly at the house, but it was rarely a kid asking for Daniel to come out and play. If he did join, it often didn't last long, and he'd stomp back into the house and complain about how unfair some of the kids were and how they just wouldn't listen.

As a fifth grader, Daniel wanted to play with the other kids, but they often found him annoying and said that he didn't always like doing the things they liked. He wasn't riding a bike yet, so there were times when he couldn't keep up. While Daniel typically did well in school, his parents saw the amount of redirection that was required to do his work during the pandemic and how frequently his frustration would result in a major blowup.

Daniel's Brain Balance assessment revealed many things, with the most significant areas showing issues with balance, proprioception, several primitive reflexes, and coordinated eye movements. He was a brilliant kid with an amazing memory, but many elements of development were lagging, making it harder for him to sustain focus, control his temper when he was frustrated with peers or parents, and interact with others. The result was a kid who felt like nobody liked him. He spent more time gaming by himself and less time moving and interacting with other kids and the world, which was not helping his development.

Fast-forward several months after working on Daniel's foundations of development. He told me one of the best things I've ever heard: "I know my brain's getting stronger because I don't annoy people as much anymore. When someone tells me to knock it off, I can now. Sometimes I even know they're getting annoyed before they say it!"

He went on to say that he used to know he was annoying people when they told him, but he couldn't help it and didn't always know what he did that annoyed them.

There's nothing better than hearing what the kids notice themselves and hearing it in their own words! Daniel's mom said she knew things were getting better when the neighbor kids started asking for him when they came to the door—day after day.

Verbal communication is another key element to building relationships and socializing, but how do you get your child to move beyond the one- or two-word answers?

"How was your day?"

"Fine."

"How did the history test go?"

"Dunno."

"What did you have for lunch today?"

"Can't remember."

If conversations with your kids ever sound like that, this section is for you.

Earlier, I mentioned how many separate brain networks must all work together for communication, and we've also talked about the brain's need for rest and fuel to function well. But it's easy to forget those details when you haven't seen your kid all day, and you're picking them up from school and want to catch up.

One of the biggest keys to successful communication with your child—at any age—is timing. And the timing isn't about what works for *you* but what works for *them*.

Communication pathways take energy, and kids haven't had as many years to use those pathways as we have. Which means it takes more energy and effort for them, especially if you're asking them to retrieve information from their memory ("What did you eat for lunch at school?") or think before they respond (rather than blurting out something that may be unkind, or not appropriate to be said).

By the end of a school day, kids are usually depleted in both energy and resources. They often come home hungry, tired, and even irritable.

To create an environment that supports conversation, approach them after they've eaten and are energized. Ideally, wait twenty minutes after they've had a protein snack. It's smart to wait to chat until after they've rested or after they've exercised, since both activities help to re-engage the brain. Then practice. The more they use those communication pathways, the greater ease in engaging they will have over time.

Relationship and Social Development Activities for Elementary School Students

Activities to support proprioception
Balance activities:
- Use the balance beam
- Rollerblade
- Ice skate
- Jump on a trampoline
- Skateboard
- Ride a scooter
- Jump on a pogo stick

Body awareness and movement activities:
- Play charades
- Play freeze tag
- Do agility ladder exercises

- Play hopscotch
- Do martial arts
- Practice yoga
- Dance
- Play a two-point discrimination game: Have your child sit with their eyes closed. Tap your child on two body parts, then ask them to raise the body part you tapped. For example, when you tap their right knee and left hand, they should raise both parts. They need to process what they feel, then respond by moving the corresponding part. Once they've mastered that, increase the difficulty by using your words instead of tapping. Say, "Right hand, left elbow. Left foot, left hand. Right knee, turn head to the left." They'll need to process the information, then coordinate the correct body part to respond.

Activities to support communication:
- Role-play examples of scenarios and actions. Be playful and have fun. Exaggerate the examples and responses to help support your point. You can role-play any upset or scenario that could've been handled differently: asking to take a turn rather than butting in to a game, listening to what someone is saying instead of interrupting, answering a question but in a kind tone rather than a rude tone. Role-play at a time when everyone's in a good mood and is cooperative—not in the middle of an upset. Now, you do the role play and ask your child to point out what you should do differently next time—or what was good about how you responded. Have your child act out good/bad examples of how to handle an upset.
- Use car time to practice communication.
  - Story chain: start a story that the next person continues. For example, the first person starts the story, "Once upon a time in the desert there lived a bunny . . ." Then the next person must pick up the story where it left off, "and that bunny was no ordinary bunny . . ."
  - Rapid-fire brainstorming:
    - Quickly list as many types of cars, cereal, animals, states, cities, and so on as you can in one minute

- List one animal that begins with each letter of the alphabet
- Give a word, then think of all the different words you could use to describe the same thing. For example: mad = angry, upset, irritated
- Point out examples of emotions, expressions, and behavior. "Right now I'm so tired and frustrated. Do you see my frustrated face and my exhausted posture? How else can you tell I'm tired?" or "I notice that you seem excited and happy right now. I can tell because you have a huge smile on your face, and you're very animated and lively with your voice and body as you're talking."

Middle School and High School Students

Throughout the teen years priorities will continue to shift, with kids placing greater importance on friendships and peer dynamics. A focus on building a sense of community and belonging with a greater sense of independence from family can create a challenging dynamic at home. To me these years have felt a bit like fishing—casting the kids out and reeling them back in over and over as they build confidence and awareness of their place in the world. Friendships, romantic interests, and social dynamics are a big influence, and their emotions can feel extreme as they face many experiences for the first time.

Relationship and Social Development Milestones
for Middle School and High School Students

Thirteen to fourteen years:[22]
- Takes on more responsibility at home
- Takes responsibility for homework with little prodding
- Is socially expansive and aware
- Can be inconsistent and unpredictable
- Is competitive and wants to excel
- Shows extremes of emotions
- Enjoys close interactions with peers, especially same gender
- Has inadequate coping skills to handle stress and challenges alone

- Wants immediate gratification
- Can recognize personal strengths and challenges
- Is embarrassed by family and parents
- May seem self-centered, impulsive, or moody
- Is eager to be accepted by peers and have friends

Fifteen to eighteen years:[23]

- Doesn't want to talk as much
- Can be argumentative
- May appreciate siblings more than parents
- Narrows down to a few close friends and may start dating
- Analyzes their own feelings and tries to find the cause of them
- Has more romantic interests
- Goes through less conflict with parents
- Shows more independence from parents
- Has deeper capacity for caring and sharing and for developing more intimate relationships
- Spends less time with parents and more time with friends
- Feels a lot of sadness or depression, which can lead to poor grades at school, alcohol and drug use, unsafe sex, and other problems
- Starts relating to family
- Begins to see parents as real people
- Develops a better sense of who they are and what positive things they can contribute to friendships and relationships
- Is able to voice emotions to try to find solutions to conflicts[24]

Everybody needs somebody. But for some kids, finding their people or person may be harder than it is for others. Stella struggled to fit in throughout middle school, and then school shut down due to COVID. When students finally returned, everyone went back wearing masks, which, along with the limited activities and time for interactions, made it even harder. The result was several hard years for both Stella and her parents, who watched her struggle but didn't know how to help.

Stella had never been a *sporty* kid, as her mom described it, and after trying sport after sport and living through those frustrations, it was clear these weren't her thing. Her parents pushed her toward soccer, dance, gymnastics, and a church youth group but didn't know what would help her make connections with friends. Complicating things further, Stella's older sister was both athletic and outgoing and made friends easily wherever she went.

Stella dreaded entering high school with its larger building, new kids and teachers, and what seemed inevitable: more time feeling like the odd one out. But Stella was quickly—and pleasantly—surprised that in high school, there were so many more options for sports, clubs, and activities. In the first month, Stella signed up for several clubs and came home one day and declared to her mom, "I've found my people!" She joined the theater club and an anime sketch club ("Who knew there was such a thing?"), and she found other kids with similar interests. The clubs pulled together groups of kids and provided them with activities that broke the ice and formed connections.

Finding high school clubs that Stella liked sparked some additional ideas of things she might enjoy with kids outside of school, and after making new friends through the clubs, she now had friends to spend time with both in school and outside of school.

While the middle school and high school years are important for social interactions and learning, the middle school years, by nature, are a time when kids focus on themselves, the need to fit in, and their sense of belonging with peers. This need continues beyond middle school, but is heightened at this time as kids are branching out from the security of home and family and looking to peer groups to help define who they are as a person and where they feel they fit in. The pandemic made this even harder for our teens. Further complicating things is social media, which only amplifies the fixation and focus on self. A study published in 2020 found that rates of narcissism, self-promotion, and antisocial behavior in teens had sharply increased over the past decade, attributed in part to social media usage.[25] And that was *before* the pandemic, when screen time for many kids doubled compared to pre-pandemic rates.[26]

A study published in 2021 from a team of researchers out of the University of Missouri–Columbia found that happiness increases when you're focused on making others feel happy rather than yourself. Helping others is one of the best ways to make ourselves feel good.[27] The researchers shared that feelings of relatedness or being close to others may help explain why helping others boosts our own mood. The study also found that while connection to other people was a contributing factor, doing anonymous good deeds for others—such as feeding a parking meter for a stranger—still created positive feelings.

This point was driven home in a recent conversation with a friend about their family's summer adventures. While their summer was filled with camps and travel, for her middle son, Noah, his favorite part of summer was a week he spent volunteering in Kentucky. He worked with the organization Appalachia Service Project, whose mission is to deliver home repairs for families in need throughout the region with volunteer labor and supplies. The week is a hard one—sleeping on cots in school gymnasiums and doing physical labor all day in the heat and humidity. But you also spend time with the families whose homes you are helping to build or repair. The families invite you into their homes as guests that week, sharing meals and stories. I was fortunate to have been involved with this program each summer throughout high school, and again as an adult volunteer leading a team of youth years later. Hearing about Noah's experience brought back happy and vivid memories of the homes and families we worked with and the team of peers I worked alongside as we patched and painted, repaired roofs, and installed plumbing (with lots of help). Like Noah, this hard work helping others was a summer highlight of mine for years.

Encouraging our teens to think beyond their own needs can help them engage and connect with the world around them, shifting their focus from *self* to *others*. There are ways to do this in simple everyday actions and habits, as well as intentional plans and experiences that can both broaden their horizons and create awareness of the world and others.

- Encourage them to be a good friend and work through what it means to be a good friend in words, actions, and deeds.
- Help your teens be aware of the kind and thoughtful actions of others and how they impact your teen.
- Create a home culture of kindness and thoughtfulness with a focus on how that impacts other people.

I learned a great example of expressing thoughtfulness from a family I knew through Brain Balance years ago. This family takes one day each year to deliver small gifts to an entire list of people. Their goal is to put a smile on the recipient's face and to let them know that even if they don't see them often, they think of them and are thankful for them. One year, I was an unexpected recipient of this simple gesture, and nearly ten years later I still remember the beautiful flowering plant and the fact that they went out of their way to make me smile.

The mom shared that over the years, the kids have gotten more and more into planning out the lists, gestures, and surprises—to the point where they began doing it more than once a year.

They experience as much joy themselves throughout the year as they plan and make their lists as when they deliver the gifts. And they've found additional joy in watching their act of thoughtfulness spread as other families have started similar traditions. This family created a way for their kids to think and act with a continual focus on kindness and bringing joy to others.

Having positive relationships and connections with peers takes awareness of others and an ability to engage and interact. And social media can hinder those interactions if not kept in check.

One approach to shift the focus from inward to outward is to work toward creating balance regarding social media usage. Social media has good elements as well as bad, and since it doesn't appear to be going away anytime soon, learning to live with it with a healthy balance and awareness is a more effective long-term strategy than fighting it.

Talk with your kids about what you see in your own social media accounts and how it makes you feel as well as the difference between a photo and real life. When you see someone post about their travel, it can make you wish you could plan a trip like that, and suddenly you're less excited about your own spring break plans. Seeing people you enjoy in a picture together when you're not there can make you feel left out. Seeing the influencers modeling summer dresses, or the targeted ads of clothes or jewelry, can constantly tempt you to purchase new outfits. And the filtered and airbrushed pictures of perfection can make you more insecure about your own looks. If your kids are already feeling down or in a bad mood, time on social media is more likely to amplify the bad mood, not reverse it.

Scrolling social media when they need to focus or study pulls attention away from learning, makes that time less productive, and burns through fuel resources. Save the social media time as a reward for when they've finished studying.

Before your kids grab their phone to start scrolling, encourage them to ask themselves a few questions:

1. **How am I feeling right now?** If you're feeling anything other than happy and fulfilled, set it aside!
2. **Is there anything I should be doing with my time right now?** Using the phone to procrastinate will only increase stress. Save it until after you're done, then relax and enjoy a little downtime.
3. **What am I trying to accomplish by posting or going online?** If you're trying to see what someone else is doing, or trying to prove a point through your post, set it aside. Nothing good or positive will come from those actions.

If your kids enjoy posting on social media, think of strategies to guide their posts and social media usage in a healthy direction.

- Discuss how they can create a message by being thoughtful in their posts and topics, rather than focusing on selfies and superficial subjects such as new clothes or their appearance.
- Do you love nature? Selecting images that show examples of what you love about nature, or of yourself enjoying nature, can shift the focus from *me* to *something I love*—a slight yet meaningful difference.
- Love sports? Share images of the hard work that goes into excelling at a sport and the people you admire because of what they've contributed to the sport.
- Teach your kids to put thought behind their posts and to emphasize the message they want to share with the world—the world that includes family, friends, future employers, and universities.

- Make recommendations on a time limit. Use the screen time limits in the phone or an outside app to monitor and control usage. You can also have your kids set a timer on their phone with a noise notification to prevent falling down the black hole when scrolling.
- Be accountability buddies with your kids when using social media. We could all adopt healthier habits, and by working together to talk about how you feel and being aware of your actions and time, it can help everyone learn and grow in positive ways.

Relationship and Social Development Activities for Middle School and High School Students

- Encourage your child to get involved in any activity that involves other kids the same age. While sports are fantastic for so many reasons, think beyond sports. Explore classes and activities through your local community center, community colleges, local universities, meet-up groups, religious youth groups, and theater and arts organizations.
- To help your kids think beyond themselves, have them volunteer at a daycare, a special needs care, the local food pantry, an elder care facility, or a local race. The opportunities are endless. Contact your local chamber of commerce if you need ideas specific to your area.
- Practice social media balance. It takes awareness and discipline— which means trial, error, and time—to learn to balance social media usage and to understand when is the best time to engage in it.
  - Start by keeping a social media journal. Do this as a family to increase everyone's awareness. Record the metrics your phone tracks—total screen usage, time by app, number of times you pick up your phone per day.
  - Next, write down one or two words that summarize your mood and then continue tracking your usage.
  - Finally, as a family, map out a plan. When are good times to use social media and for how long? Ideal times are after all work and chores have been completed, when you're in a good mood, and for only thirty minutes at a time.

Signs That Indicate Improvement

As your child's social and communication abilities begin to improve, you may find yourself thinking, "They seem older now, more mature." Their actions and interactions will begin to be more age appropriate (even if age-appropriate behavior is silly behavior, pushing boundaries, or pushing back against parents). You'll even notice their interests and activities evolve as they mature in their development. Remember that each stage of development comes with both positive and challenging behaviors as kids strive toward autonomy and independence, relying more on friends over time than parents. It will begin with small things: eye contact, more than a one-word answer, an increase in social ease and comfort, less anxiety and worrying. When it comes to improved awareness of nonverbal communication involving body language, they'll initially notice it but won't know what it means. Over time you may begin to notice a change in how your child interprets sarcasm and humor if this was something they previously struggled to grasp. You can experience a shift or evolution in conversations with your child, with more back-and-forth and a greater depth to the topics and discussions. At first, they'll take everything personally, then as their catalogue of understanding improves, they'll begin to better interpret the cues and won't default to thinking everything is against them. When those moments of hurt feelings or confusion occur, remember that this is a part of the development process and can provide great opportunities for learning and conversations.

You'll know your child is at a great place regarding relationships, awareness, and communication when they can identify and then communicate how they're feeling or doing and can recognize and react to emotions and needs in others. Be sure to listen when this happens to continue to encourage and support this level of engagement as they interact and build fulfilling friendships in their life!

6

. . . .

LEARNING

Learning can be such a fun and even inspiring experience when you're learning about a topic that excites and motivates you or a concept finally clicks into place. **In fact, dopamine, the feel-good chemical we discussed in chapter 4, is released when learning something new and interesting, signaling to the brain that something good and rewarding just happened.**[1] The dopamine release can leave you feeling invigorated, encouraging you to want to continue to learn so as to elicit that same feeling time and time again. Studying hard then acing a test or getting an answer correct in class feels good because of the brain's response. These are all moments that contribute to a child's sense of self and understanding of what they are capable of accomplishing. But there's another side to learning that can be arduous and disheartening. Studying for hours and failing a test, not being able to keep up, no matter how hard you try, feeling like a disappointment to yourself and others makes it hard to want to continue the effort when the results are less than desirable. When learning isn't going well, mood, emotions, and behaviors can all be impacted. Dopamine has also been shown to help your brain decide if the challenge is worth the effort, to guide behaviors and decisions.[2]

Note to Parents

Nobody likes doing things that are hard for them, so if your typically easy-going kid starts acting up when learning or homework is mentioned, watch closely. The distractions and antics will vary by age, but the theme remains the same—they are trying to avoid a task that's difficult.

When it comes to learning, there are several red flags that indicate your child is struggling—and sometimes that struggle can be directly related to their development. Indicators of challenges include: grades or test scores that drop or are inconsistent; homework time lasting longer for them than for their classmates (if you're not sure about this, talk to their teacher to get a sense of how long the homework should be taking); a need for more repetition for new concepts to make sense; or a change in mood and behaviors when it's time to learn. The trick is digging deeper to understand *where* the challenge is coming from to determine the most efficient and effective way to support their learning, work, and outcomes.

Younger kids will often get silly or upset; melt down; decide they are hungry, thirsty, or need the bathroom; or all of the above. Older students may procrastinate, become irritable or belligerent, or just shut down. **Regardless of age, feeling overwhelmed happens when you don't feel you have the resources—the knowledge, the time, or the ability—to do what is asked of you, to complete the task or project.** Kids may lie about the work they have been assigned or hide their work to avoid it—and to avoid the effort and discomfort that comes from doing something they don't feel equipped to do. The consistent element across the ages is that kids (and adults) will do anything and everything they can to avoid or procrastinate on tasks that aren't fun. And it's never fun when you don't understand the directions, the assignment, or the content itself.

We know that kids fell behind in many aspects during the pandemic. This was demonstrated by the results of the 2022 National Assessment of Educational Progress, a standardized test that is used to measure student achievement in nine-year-olds, following the COVID-19 period of distance learning. The data showed the largest decline in mathematics scores since the test began in 1969, and the largest decline in reading in three decades.[3] This leaves both schools and families around the world scrambling to support their kids' education. The curriculum standards and expectations for achievement going forward have not been modified as a result of these demonstrated gaps, which means the expectations are the same, but the kids are starting from a lower point, increasing the stress and burden on students, teachers, and parents.

Whether or not your child is struggling academically, in this chapter I hope to arm you with information and a plan to help optimize your child's learning experience by supporting and enhancing their development. When the brain is taking in, processing, and reacting to information optimally, learning can be a lifelong source of interest and fulfillment. Knowing how to support your child's specific needs is the key to ensuring a positive learning experience.

Pandemic Lessons

"Virtual learning is virtually no education at all."[4] Headlines and quotes such as this one in the *Baltimore Sun* filled the news for over two years, as we realized more and more just how far our kids were falling behind academically at all ages. Like all of us, our schools scrambled to put a new plan in place overnight, but it was a plan that left far too many kids without the necessary access, scaffolding, and oversight needed to ensure engagement and mastery of concepts. The strategy of virtual learning resulted in kids falling behind, with students in single-parent households and lower socioeconomic regions left even further behind, widening the existing achievement gap.

While schools did the best they could to scramble and deliver remote instruction, studies indicate substantially less learning occurred with the virtual workarounds. A study in the Netherlands indicated that "despite favorable conditions, we find that students made little or no progress while learning from home." A drop in completed work, a decline in student attendance, and a larger difference between the low and high test scores were all early indicators that learning was not on a good course.[5]

Data analysis of 5.4 million U.S. kids in third through eighth grades demonstrated that while gains were made during the 2020–2021 school year, those gains were smaller than in previous years, smaller for math than reading, and even smaller in low socioeconomic schools.[6] COVID revealed many inequities and disproportionately hurt low-income students, students with special needs, and underresourced schools. An article from the *Harvard Gazette*, "How COVID Taught America about Inequity in Education," points out the degree of racial inequity. As one example, it noted that "Black and Hispanic households with school-aged children were 1.3 to 1.4 times as likely as white ones to face limited access to computers and the internet."[7]

Early elementary students have shown larger decreases in reading skills than older students, with a 2022 *New York Times* article reporting that one-third of children in the earliest grades are missing reading benchmarks, up significantly compared to pre-pandemic levels.[8] A study from the University of Virginia's School of Education and Human Development found reading levels were at a twenty-year low, which researchers described as "alarming,"[9] and a Boston school quoted in the *New York Times* piece shared that 60% of students at some high-poverty schools have been identified as being at high risk for reading problems, double the previous levels.

Kids are back in class but are facing the newly widened achievement gap and increased issues in the classroom. These issues include a wide range of challenges, from an increase in mental health concerns, which can interfere with attention and learning, to higher rates of violence and misbehaviors.[10] Layered on top of those challenges are national teacher shortages. Teaching has never been an easy job, and the past few years have only made it harder.

For many students, catching up academically will simply require exposure to or review of the material that was missed. But for some kids returning to the classroom, a review of the material may not be enough.

From infants to kids of all grades, there was a disruption in the formative development that is critical for evolving the *ability* to learn—cognition. Remember the definition of *cognition?* The mental access or process of acquiring knowledge and understanding through thought, experience, and the senses. The pandemic disrupted the development of cognition, leaving kids further behind in their knowledge, experiences, and senses, as well as in their exposure to material. How could they not fall behind?

Many of the individual brain functions we discuss in this book contribute to learning—sensory perception, attention, and memory all must work together to create comprehension. And while schools and parents typically have a big focus on the "what" of learning—the content—there is far less focus and understanding on the elements that contribute to the "how"— how you take in, organize, store, and retrieve information so that you can utilize knowledge not only for school requirements such as homework and tests but also for life in general. Beyond a learning style or strategy, the brain needs networks that coordinate to facilitate learning.

Science Alert

Learning is defined as the acquisition of knowledge and skills through experience, study, or instruction. But what this definition doesn't take into consideration is all that is required of the brain in the process of learning and the many separate networks and hubs in the brain that must fire simultaneously to succeed.

First, the learner must have the ability to direct and sustain their attention—you can't remember what you don't see or hear. But attention is not the full story: a recent study looking at ADHD medication and learning demonstrated that attention alone isn't enough for learning. This study found that kids on medication saw an increase in attention, self-regulation impacting behavior, and seated work time, but found "little detectable impact on how much a child with attention deficit hyperactivity disorder learns in the classroom."[11] **Attention contributes to learning but isn't the full story in creating learning success.**

Next, the learner must accurately process the information—this requires precise perception of what the eyes see and the ears hear. It is key to note that studies have indicated a correlation in sensory processing and dyslexia, a condition with which individuals may struggle to read as well as to discern speech in a noisy environment. A study published in the science journal *Neuron* indicated that in healthy development the brain rapidly adapts to the changing sensory input we hear and see to make processing this information more efficient. In individuals diagnosed with dyslexia, their adaptation was on average half of those without the condition.[12]

After paying attention and processing, the learner must store the new knowledge in their memory so it can be applied at the correct time and in the right context. Disruptions in attention, memory, and sensory processing can disrupt absorption of content. And that's just the beginning. A person's mood and energy can also play a role in their learning—depression, anxiety, worries, and fatigue are all things that can decrease attention, memory, and cognition, ultimately making learning even harder.

Learning is complex and is about so much more than the content itself. When you start to break down all the separate neural networks and skills that contribute to learning, it's mind-boggling and makes you realize how truly amazing it is that any of us learn and retain anything at all.

Now for the good news: the brain *loves* to learn. When you learn something that interests or motivates you, or moves you closer to achieving a goal, it generates positive emotions by releasing dopamine, the "feel good" neuro-transmitter mentioned earlier. Think about the last time you learned something that excited you—you wanted to share it with others; it gave you energy! It's why listening to an informative podcast or attending a seminar as an adult is so rewarding (or can be, given the right topic that interests you).

Disruptions or challenges in any of the pathways that support learning—attention, memory, sensory processing, including auditory and visual processing—can interrupt learning, resulting in a frustrating experience. All too often, when someone is struggling with learning, the approach to review the material falls short or completely misses the mark of what is needed for that student.

Before you spend more time reviewing the same content, it is helpful to consider the types of pathways and functions that support learning. By making sure that the brain has the capacity to support aspects of cognition through mature connections and timing, you can set the learner up for a more successful experience.

Reading is a great example of how many separate networks in the brain must all come online at the same time to result in successful comprehension. The reader must understand phonics to sound out each letter in a word. There is also word analysis—the ability to understand the meaning of parts of a word to contribute to understanding the meaning of a word. Memory contributes to sight words so that a reader doesn't need to decode a word each time it is presented. Visual tracking allows the eyes to move through a word and then move across a line of text and on to the next line of text. Visual processing allows the brain to understand what the eyes are seeing. Each of these skills relies on separate networks in the brain, while additional networks that support reading comprehension also contribute simultaneously.

Separate networks working together form hubs in the brain. These hubs are considered key to brain communication and neural integration.[13] Nearly all cognitive functions require different hubs—the combination of separate tasks coalescing (the scientific term for this is *dynamic coupling*—referring to separate networks firing together). Recent research indicates that brain hubs play important roles in information integration "across numerous aspects of complex cognitive function."[14] Scientists from the University of Cambridge found that connectivity related to hubs plays a key role in learning. The study found that kids with poorly connected brain hubs had widespread cognitive difficulties impacting learning.[15]

Helping your child address the mechanics that guide learning can be a great strategy to build confidence and knowledge—and find the joy in education. This will also contribute to supporting long-term mental well-being by keeping the brain active, engaged, and thriving.

Providing our kids with rich sensory exposure and experiences helps to build pathways to support learning. Finding ways for new and different experiences and opportunities to move, play, and increase coordination and timing leads to more complex development, improving our abilities to succeed with attention, memory, comprehension, prediction, planning, and execution. We simply can't sacrifice time spent strengthening the pathways that create the foundation for skills to grow and improve. All kids, and especially the pandemic generation, need *both* academic practice and support of their cognitive neural development.

Infants and Toddlers

While learning is a lifelong pursuit, the amount of learning that takes place in the early years is mind-boggling. An infant's brain has more connections at age two than the adult brain does. Then, over time, through use the brain prunes the connections, prioritizing what is deemed most important. The CDC emphasizes the importance of early childhood experiences for brain development and considers the first eight years foundational for future learning.[16]

Learning Development Milestones for Infants and Toddlers

Zero to two years:[17]

- Learn by exploring with their hands—banging, throwing, dropping, and shaking—and by putting items in their mouths

- Smile and giggle when they want more of something
- Turn their head away or cry when they want less of something
- Respond to changes in other people's behaviors, facial expressions, and emotions

Two years: [18]

- Knows around fifty words
- Is able to point to at least two body parts when you ask them
- Can name objects in a book when you point
- Uses things to pretend; for example, feeds a block to a doll as if it were food
- Shows simple problem-solving skills, like standing on a small stool to reach something
- Follows two-step directions like "put the toy down and close the door"
- Knows at least one color; for example, can answer "which one is red?" when looking at crayons

Three years: [19]

- Knows around 300 words
- Imaginary play contributes to intellectual development
- Understands and avoids touching hot objects like a stove

Four years: [20]

- Knows around 1,500 words
- Names a few colors
- Can do simple counting
- Tells what comes next in a familiar story
- Draws a person with three or more body parts
- During these preschool years is learning to cooperate, solve problems, and share

Learning is a lifelong process that begins in infancy and hopefully never ends. For infants, learning begins by engaging with their environment and the people that surround them. **Learning happens through the senses and will be practiced through engagement and repetition—trial, error, and play.** [21] Each new tidbit learned forms a new connection in the brain. Then reviewing that information engages and strengthens that pathway, making it faster and easier to access. To support your infant or toddler's learning, engage as many of the senses as possible. Sight, sound, touch, smell, and perception of movement will exercise and engage networks that provide information, and all contribute to learning. In fact, research shows that the senses can enhance memory and that the regions in the brain that process smells and memories are in close proximity.[22] Have you ever noticed how a particular smell can trigger a vivid memory? Instant memories and feelings are evoked from the smell of your grandmother's perfume, for instance—a scent you recognize even though you may not know the name. All because of the power of your senses and memory.

Preschools understand the importance of sensory play and provide a combination of experiences, from outside playtime to songs, arts, crafts, and more. My son Drew's class would also incorporate smell and taste occasionally. One example of this created Drew's most vivid preschool memory.

I knew something had gone awry on this day when at pickup his normally polished and lovely teachers were not in their usual calm and collected state. To say there was a sense of disruption is an understatement. One teacher's hair was disheveled, several kids had on wet shirts, and the room was in disarray.

"Everything okay?" I asked Drew's lead teacher under my breath, in case it wasn't something they wanted to share in front of the kids or other parents.

"Chain-reaction puking," was the answer I got.

What started as quiet circle time to touch, smell, and taste various foods went downhill quickly when one of the girls tasted dark chocolate powder for the first time. She smelled it, tasted it, then instantly gagged and puked. This resulted in three more kids puking. "It just didn't stop," the teacher confided.

To this day it is still one of Drew's favorite stories to tell from preschool. Thankfully, he was not one of the pukers; however, the memory is still a strong one. This experience provided a new and different experience for the kids, and not just from tasting the dark chocolate but from the sights, sounds, and smells that happened next (ew!). The senses are a powerful component of learning and memory.

While I hope you can avoid this particular experience, the takeaway message is that by engaging as many of the senses as you can in new experiences, you are increasing the likelihood that your child will retain the experience in their long-term memory to be applied to future situations.

Next, focus on repetition. Repetition. Repetition. Each time you repeat a thought, action, or reaction, you engage the same neurological connections in the brain, leading to more efficient pathways. The scientific journal *Frontiers for Young Minds* describes learning by stating, "When you are learning, important changes take place in the brain, including the creating of new connections between your neurons. This phenomenon is called neuroplasticity. The more you practice, the stronger these connections become. As your connections strengthen, the messages (nerve impulses) are transmitted increasingly faster, making them more efficient."[23]

From physical coordination to sight words to memorizing a math formula—it is all specific connections in the brain coordinating with precise timing. Repetition makes these connections more permanent, so they can be used at any time—now or ten years from now if they have been strengthened enough. If you've heard the term "muscle memory" then you get it—a movement you can do with ease is an example of a set pattern of neurons firing, working together as a specific network to carry out a specific action. This applies to not just movements but thoughts, behaviors, and the learning of new information as well.

Kids love repetition. The brain naturally seeks the practice and reinforcement that will result in learning. Repetition is familiar, and familiar is comfortable to kids.

Think back to bedtime stories with your kids. How many times did you read *Go, Dog. Go!* or *The Little Engine That Could*? While you may have been bored out of your mind reading that same book for the hundredth time, your kids found joy in the routine, in knowing what to expect, in looking for the same pictures they loved or the sounds they found funny. They were strengthening the pathways in their brain, which allowed them to understand the story. Utilizing this knowledge can help to reframe your annoyance in rereading those familiar books and can support learning and familiarity with other things as well.

Finding ways to create repetition and routines—even with babies too young to fully comprehend what you're doing—can be beneficial. You can count while doing everyday tasks—while getting your baby dressed, say, "one arm, two arms" as you are putting on their shirt. Walking up stairs, count "one . . . two . . . three!" Kids will memorize and repeat what you say before they understand that the word you are saying represents a number of items. Over time they will start to correlate those memorized words with their meanings.

As parents it is way too easy to get distracted, become overwhelmed, and function on autopilot. It is often a survival mechanism. When you catch yourself operating this way, take a step back and regroup. How can you maximize some of the opportunities available right now to connect with and actively support your kids' learning and development?

We've all heard of "hands-on learning," but we can take that concept even further to engage and exercise the brain: hands-on, feet-on, whole-body learning. By adding movement and engaging multiple senses, you will engage even more networks and pathways in the brain simultaneously. Engaging large regions of the brain through motion and movement to help create memories is called *kinesthetic learning*—adding movement to enhance learning.

While adding movement to learning can feel strange at first, with awareness and practice it will begin to feel much more natural. Start by simply adding vocab practice to the things your child is already doing while moving. When you're at the park and your child is climbing, talk about what they are doing. "Up! You're climbing up the ladder!" "Down! You're sliding down the slide!" *Big, small, over, under*—there are endless opportunities for vocabulary development in this environment. While not everything in life needs to be a lesson, working learning into play makes it fun and easy to do.

You can also add movement to other things you're helping your child learn. And the movement doesn't need to have anything to do with what you're teaching. If your child is beginning to learn colors, make it a game to clap every time you see something red while riding in the car. Then, once they have that down, add a second color and movement. For example, stomp every time you see an object in the shape of a square.

While this can feel awkward at first, the more you do it, the more natural it will become, and it can help to instill a powerful lifelong learning strategy for your child.

Learning Development Activities for Infants and Toddlers

- Layer sensory stimulation: Sing about what you are doing while playing with the gritty texture of sand, the cold water in the sink, the smooth, fluffy texture of shaving cream.
- Draw shapes as part of sensory play: Draw a circle in shaving cream while saying the shape, noticing the color, and smelling the shaving cream—touch, sound, sight, smell
- Include repetition: Repetition is key to learning, so playing the same games over and over, reading the same books, listening to the same songs, and telling the same stories is not only helpful but needed. There are many ways you can create repetition. The following are examples of creating patterns and routines by saying or singing the same phrase throughout the day:
  - Sing your child's name to the tune of the Mickey Mouse Clubhouse song, "M-o-r-g-a-n."
  - Chant "one arm, two arms" while putting on a jacket.
  - Count the stairs while walking up or down: "We're going up! One, two, three stairs to the door."
- Utilize a few minutes at bedtime for learning. Tell a story each night like you are telling it for the first time: "This is a circle, circles are round and smooth. What circles can we find in your room? The clock, the picture in the book, the top of your sippy cup are all circles." Once your child can point out the circles in their room, change the directions, and you can point to an object for your child to name. "What shape is the clock on the wall?"
- Let your little ones explore cause and effect through repetition as well.
  - Let them drop their sippy cup on the floor over and over when they're sitting in their high chair. This shows them what happens when they drop something. It falls, and you come to pick it back up.

○ Provide a bin of toys they can dump out (then sing the cleanup song together as you put the toys back in the bin to do it all over again).

○ Play peekaboo or hide a Cheerio in your hand and have them guess which hand has the Cheerio. This helps kids learn object permanence, the understanding that something is still there even though they can't see it.

• Add movement to learning—car time is a great time to do this since it keeps the kids entertained without technology. Wave your hands in the air each time you see the letter B, or clap every time you hear the "B" sound (or anything else you are working on learning).

Elementary School Students

The early elementary years are an exciting time of foundational academic learning. Watching your child begin to make sense of letters to form words as they begin to read and recognize numbers and math concepts is exciting, as it allows them to interact with the world around them in a new way.

While our schools here in the United States have a large focus on academic rigor, we can't forget the importance of learning through play and movement. The senses, repetition, and peer interactions all contribute in meaningful ways to your child's continued learning.

Learning Development Milestones for
Elementary School Students

Five years:[24]

• Counts to ten
• Names some numbers between one and five when you point to them
• Uses words about time, like *yesterday, tomorrow, morning,* or *night*
• Writes some letters in their name
• Names some letters when you point to them

Five to six years:[25]

• Speech is grammatically correct, most of the time
• Understands opposites: big/little, hard/soft, heavy/light, and so on
• Understands three commands given without interruptions

- Understands concept of time: morning, noon, night, day, later, yesterday
- Properly names primary colors and possibly many more
- Questions more deeply, addresses meaning and purpose of what you are doing and why (for example, why do I make my bed if I crawl into it again soon for bedtime?)

Six to seven years:[26]

- Has the ability to describe experiences
- Talks about thoughts and feelings
- Can tell a complicated story
- Understands relationships between objects and occurrences (for example, when I push the truck down a hill it will roll away quickly)
- Knows left hand from right hand
- Can repeat three numbers backward
- Can read age-appropriate books

Seven to eight years:[27]

- Tells time to the quarter hour using an analog clock
- Begins to reason and concentrate
- Has a solid sense of time: seconds, minutes, hours, days, weeks, months, seasons, years
- Solves simple math problems using objects (such as counting beads)
- Performs at grade level in all subjects

Eight to nine years:[28]

- May develop a major interest in reading
- Displays organized and logical thinking
- Recognizes the concept of reversibility ($4 + 2 = 6$ and $6 - 2 = 4$)
- Knows what day of the week it is
- Has a black-and-white perspective much of the time (impacting perception of right/wrong, fair/unfair, etc.)
- Can count backward
- Understands fractions

Nine to ten years:[29]

- Follows fairly complex directions with little repetition
- Has well-developed concepts of time and numbers

- Can think independently and clearly (but thinking is tied to what their friends think)
- Is beginning to make decisions

Ten to eleven years:[30]

- Solves abstract problems using logic
- Displays concrete, rational, and logical skills
- Has an accurate perception of events
- Possesses a surprising scope of interests
- Is eager to master new skills
- Writes stories

Elementary school is a critical time for both academic and social/emotional learning, as everything builds on the skills developed during these years. Starting with the basics, early elementary learning relies heavily on memory—students must learn numbers, letters, phonics, math facts, and more. Once the basics have been established (which means there is a set pattern of brain connections that fire each time you see "red" or "2 + 2 = 4"), the curriculum shifts to adding more involved comprehension. In K–3 you learn to read, and from fourth grade on up you read to learn—history, social studies, even math all require reading comprehension. In math, students apply their memorized math facts to story problems. Memorized grammar and spelling become sentences and eventually essays.

If your child needs more repetition or support to stay on track at school, understanding the challenge and addressing it early is critical to prevent them from falling further behind. Helping your child find success in learning will also be key for instilling a positive sense of self-confidence when it comes to school and learning.

To support your child's learning, start by watching for the subtle—or not-so-subtle—clues that let you know something is hard. Think of the struggle you see as the *symptom* of their challenge, not the challenge itself. Your job is to dig deeper to understand why they are having a hard time. For example, your child hates math. Perhaps they review basic math facts repeatedly month after month but still aren't getting them. The issue isn't math; it may be working memory.

This happened to Stephanie, a friend of mine, years ago when a teacher contacted her about her daughter Olivia's reading. Stephanie had been spending several nights a week with Olivia reviewing sight words, completing worksheets, and reading together. Most nights involved arguments and frustration for both mother and daughter, but progress was being made—slowly. Eventually the teacher reached out after a school reading test showed Olivia was significantly behind.

Stephanie was upset, concerned, and frustrated. Olivia was starting to talk negatively about herself, saying things like "I'm stupid" and "this is too hard." The school was preparing to put additional services in place to spend more one-on-one time with Olivia, but Stephanie had seen firsthand that spending more time with the same approach wasn't helping. She got that reading was a concern that needed to be addressed, but she wasn't confident in the school's plan, and she didn't know what else to do to support Olivia.

When Stephanie called, she was able to walk me through her observations. "It's like each night we sit down to work on phonics and sight words, we're starting over from scratch. We'll work on just a few sounds and words each night until she has it, but then a week or even a day later we may need to back up and do it again. If she hears me say a sound, she can tell me what letter makes that sound. If I say, 'What letter does the word *bat* start with?' She can say '*b*,' but if she sees the word *bat* she freezes. I took her to the eye doctor to see if she needs glasses, but they said her vision was great."

Stephanie was on the right track with her thinking about the eyes complicating the process, but the issue wasn't how clearly Olivia could see letters up close. The challenge turned out to be a combination of low working memory and visual processing delays. Olivia's brain required more time to process what her eyes were seeing, and low working memory required her brain to need more repetition, or stronger input, for the information to be stored in long-term memory.

I'm happy to report that by working on these supporting skills—memory and visual processing—and the developmental functions that lead to these abilities (sensory processing, coordination, and timing), Olivia was able to make big gains over the spring and summer. By fall she was testing on track, consistently scoring high grades on her work. Olivia didn't need more time reviewing the same material—she needed to improve her ability to process and retain information.

Olivia isn't the only child to benefit from strengthening foundational development to impact reading. A study published in *Neuroscience and Biobehavioral Reviews* examined many studies and found sensory deficits in several categories, including how the brain processes auditory and visual sensory stimuli for those struggling to learn how to read, including dyslexia.[31] The paper states, "Learning to read requires formation of cross-sensory associations to the point that deeply encoded multisensory representations are attained." The good news is this review study also found evidence that multi-sensory training significantly improved reading.

Key Academic Areas That Require Synchronization of Many Skills

If your child is struggling with reading, math, or writing and you want to dig deeper into your child's learning and abilities, review the academic categories below to help narrow down the challenge:

Reading

Your child needs to master all of the following functions in order to read successfully, so if a student dislikes or struggles with reading, that may be due to a challenge in one of these areas. Different brain networks contribute to each academic skill, and several networks converge through hubs to complete tasks that require several skills working together:

- Phonics (auditory processing, memory)—the age-appropriate knowledge of letter names, sounds, and letter blends; provides the ability to sound out a new word
- Sight words (visual processing, memory)—common words that children recognize and do not need to sound out; when a student has memorized sight words, they do not need to continue to decode the same word each time it appears

- Reading fluency (visual processing, eye tracking, memory)—when reading a paragraph, the eyes move smoothly and consistently through the text, no jumping or skipping of words, word parts, or lines
- Reading comprehension (visual processing, memory, ability to connect content with context)—the ability to process text, understand the meaning, and apply what you already know to pull information and meaning from the text
  - Details—one aspect of reading comprehension is the ability to retain details from the text, such as names of characters, dates, numbers, and the order of events
  - Inference—an aspect of reading comprehension that requires the reader to draw a conclusion that isn't directly stated in the passage, for example, how a character is feeling or the main idea of a text

Ask your student to read out loud. Are they able to read sight words without decoding? Once they decode a new word, are they able to read the word later in the passage without needing to decode a second or third time? Do they skip words, word parts, or lines as they read? Are they able to answer questions about the passage—provide details and facts as well as the main idea and inferential responses? If they struggle to answer questions from what they read, try reading the passage to them and see how they respond. If they do better answering questions when you read the passage to them, it may be that their eye movements or processing are interfering with their comprehension.

Math

If your child struggles with math, is it related to underlying reading challenges that impact following directions and reading story problems? Or do they struggle to memorize facts and formulas, which slows them down and causes them to make mistakes? Consider the following categories to help learn more about your child's math abilities (again, different brain networks—indicated in parentheses below—contribute to each academic skill, then work together with other networks through hubs to complete more complex skills):

- Numbers (visual processing, memory)—the ability to count and to identify a number
- Math facts (visual processing, memory)—the ability to recall addition, subtraction, multiplication, and division facts with speed and accuracy
- Math comprehension (memory, ability to connect content with context)—the understanding of what a word or number represents; for example, the number three represents three objects, or the symbol = means one thing is the same as another. Math comprehension is necessary for understanding concepts, formulas, and story problems.

Writing

Putting pen to paper to share your thoughts on a topic, in a book report, or in a story requires many elements syncing together perfectly. Like other aspects of learning, a challenge in one area can derail the end goal. If your child struggles with writing, consider the following skills supported by brain networks and hubs:

- Fine motor skills for hands (proprioception of the hands, strength, coordination, sequencing)—if writing a letter or word is hard, it can feel incredibly overwhelming and challenging to write anything more, which can result in avoidance or shortcuts to answers to complete the task as quickly and painlessly as possible.
- Grammar (memory)—the structure of language: punctuation, nouns, verbs, adverbs, verb tense, and so on
- Sequencing (memory, vocab, comprehension of time)—for a sentence to make sense, it requires the correct words in the right order (correct spelling too). Written accounts must have an accurate timeline. You can't describe the plot of a movie out of order and expect someone to follow along.
- Organization (executive function)—the ability to write the main idea with supporting statements that are relevant to the main idea.
- Multi-tasking (memory, attention, comprehension of time)—some kids have the ability to say their answer out loud, but when it comes

time to write it down, it all falls apart. As they speak, listen to see if they are organized and sequential in their answer. Are their grammar and verb tenses correct? If those pieces are in place, writing may be a challenge in the brain's ability to bring online the pathways necessary to focus and write while thinking about the question or topic—a multi-tasking challenge.

As parents, having a better understanding of what is complicating learning for your child will allow you to put the right plan in place to drive change and growth. Whether the answer is spending time each evening with your child to catch them up on content they never mastered, or working to improve eye movements, processing, or attention, your time will be better spent with a concrete plan of action based on the specific challenge your child is facing.

Listening is as complex and critical to our learning experience as seeing, yet far less time in our academic curriculum and classroom learning is dedicated to understanding and developing this skill. Monica Brady-Myerov, former NPR journalist and founder of the company Listenwise, a listening comprehension curriculum, states in her book, *Listen Wise,* "Listening is a complex neurological construct that involves multiple areas in the brain. Listening triggers a variety of parts of the brain to create a 'movie in your mind.'"[32]

Research shows that you are more likely to remember something you see than something you hear.[33] And even more likely to remember something if you hear and see it simultaneously.

Our brain is bombarded with constant information and can't possibly retain all of what we encounter. Our brain filters out so much of what we hear and see, allowing our memory to retain space and energy for what the brain deems more important.

In the classroom we depend on our listening and auditory processing to follow the teacher's directions and to learn. Listening and listening comprehension are crucial to learning, yet the larger emphasis is on reading comprehension. While that is also critical, challenges with auditory processing and listening comprehension can derail a student before they even get to the point of reading for comprehension.

Success with listening relies on a series of skills. Hearing, actively listening, processing, comprehension, memory, and attention are all distinctly separate abilities that contribute to the outcome of learning. A disruption in any one of those steps can derail the outcome. *Hearing* simply refers to your ability to hear a range of tones, while *actively listening* requires you to be paying attention to the noises, speech, or conversation happening around you. *Auditory processing* is the brain's ability to interpret the sounds you are hearing, while *comprehension* allows you to understand what those sounds or words are telling you. If you are not able to process or comprehend what you are hearing, you are less likely to commit that information to memory for later use.

Physicians and schools do early screening at birth and in school to ensure hearing and vision are accurate, that there is no need for hearing aids or glasses. To me, the next step should be a processing screening. How quickly and accurately does your brain perceive what you hear and see? Delays in auditory processing mean there's a lack of consistency or lag time between the sound and your brain's interpretation of that sound. This results in gaps of what is processed. An example is a parent saying "Go outside!" to their child. The child hears "go" so they go upstairs, and the parent is left irritated. "You didn't listen to me! I told you to go outside, not upstairs!" The child did listen but was not able to *process* all that was said.

Auditory processing improves over time and with development, allowing a child to perceive more words, syllables, and sounds. While even a young child can process rapid sounds, their consistent ability to do so improves with development and practice. Disruptions in auditory processing will disrupt learning. A child learning phonics may struggle to properly correlate what they hear with what they see if what they hear is not accurate, resulting in reading challenges. A child listening to directions who hears the first part but not the last part will do what they think they were told to do but may miss a key step. The result can be a child who appears to be uncooperative, asks more questions, struggles to keep up, pays less attention, and has increased frustration and unwanted behaviors.

Clues that may indicate a challenge in auditory processing include:

- Frequently saying "what?"
- Answering questions incorrectly (they heard the question wrong and are answering what they thought they heard)
- Needing directions to be repeated
- Often getting directions wrong
- Delaying before responding when someone speaks to them
- Struggling to follow along with a conversation or simply tuning out
- Struggles with phonics and reading
- Missing details in a show or movie they are watching, or struggling to follow along with the plot or story line
- Struggling to focus with background noise
- Zoning out (working to listen when it is hard can be exhausting, so a child may just give up)
- Exhibiting increased negative behaviors
- Disliking school
- Interrupting others during conversations

Learning Development Activities for Elementary School Students

Eye tracking and control

- On a piece of paper, draw a dot in the middle and dots one inch above, below, and to either side of the center dot. Tape the paper on a wall. Have your child stand at arm's length from the wall. Keeping their eye on the center dot, have your child turn their head left, right, and center. Then up, down, and center. Next, have them shift their eyes to the top dot and repeat the pattern. Do this for each dot, a total of five times. Next, using the same dots, while still standing at arm's length, have your child keep their head still and move only their eyes, jumping from dot to dot. Left-center-right-center. Then up-center-down-center. Work up to being able to repeat this ten times.
- Have your child use their finger to point to the letter or word as they read. Each time there is punctuation, tap the page, and tap twice at

the end of the sentence. This gives the eyes a target to return to if the eyes jump around on the page and provides both sensory input and movement to bring attention to punctuation.

Active listening skills

- Discuss and practice with your child what goes into actively listening. Discuss the importance of paying attention, making eye contact, avoiding distractions, and repeating back what you heard to confirm you both heard and understood what was said.

Auditory processing

- Play the game Simon, the classic electronic game for listening and short-term memory. The original game has four primary color buttons; each lights up and makes a specific sound. The players create a pattern, and the sequence lengthens as each player remembers, repeats, and adds onto that pattern. Simon is available on Amazon, or you can download an app version for your phone. You can also simply re-create your own version by making up a pattern by tapping, clapping, and stomping.
- Listen to radio commercials and ask questions about them. Ask both detailed questions as well as main idea and inference questions: "How do you think that person was feeling?" "What do you think they will do next?"
- Create a story chain—start a story, then each person must continue the story
- For additional listening activities and understanding, I recommend Monica Brady-Myerov's book, *Listen Wise: Teach Students to Be Better Listeners.*

Middle School and High School Students

Adolescence is a time of rapid growth and development. During this time a great deal of pruning takes place in the brain, which discards unnecessary or underused neural connections while forging new connections.[34] Increased independence and a broadening world of friendships and experiences create a time of strong opinions, boundary-pushing, and social and academic learning. This is both an exciting and intense time of life when emotions and experiences feel strong. So many experiences are still new for these maturing kids, who are growing into themselves and their interests, passions, and hobbies.

Teens' abilities have increased through development and practice, but so too have the demands and expectations around time management, multi-tasking, studying, and applying what they've learned to do well in school in preparation for life after high school.

Learning Development Milestones for Middle School and High School Students

Eleven to twelve years:[35]
- Performs at or near ability in school
- Uses deductive reasoning and makes educated guesses
- Recognizes current actions have a future effect
- Develops a conscience
- Experiences feelings of stress when academics become challenging
- May challenge assumptions and solutions presented by adults

Thirteen to fourteen years:[36]
- Can apply concepts to specific examples
- Develops a focus on the future
- Can construct hypothetical solutions to a problem and evaluate which one is best
- Engages in some fantasy
- Distinguishes fact from opinion
- Anticipates the consequences of different options
- May reject goals set by others
- Develops personal interests and abilities
- Reasons through problems even in the absence of concrete events or examples

Fifteen to seventeen years:[37]
- Learns more defined work habits
- Shows more concern about future school and work plans
- Is better able to give reasons for their own choices
- Has better understanding of what is right and wrong

Grades nine to twelve:[38]

- Shows an increased ability to reason and make educated guesses
- Starts thinking more abstractly from what *is* to what *could be*
- Uses strategies to search for, use, and compare information from multiple sources
- Uses numbers in real-life situations, like calculating tax or a tip

Learning in middle school, high school, and beyond requires some serious multi-tasking abilities that rely on our executive functions. By this time it is assumed in school that the basics have been mastered, and everything becomes more layered, more complex. Time management, organization, and discipline are now expected on top of the focus, memory, and execution needed for success in academics.

For some kids, it isn't the learning itself but the ability to pull it all together, their executive functions, that holds them back. Think of Olivia with sight words and reading: practicing the same thing doesn't always solve the problem. Sometimes the challenge is a symptom of the underlying developmental gap holding back your child's ability to pull it all together and execute on a task when needed. If your child was going to be successful in turning in their homework on their own they'd be there by now—they've had *years* of practice by this age. If there is a struggle with executive functions, exercising and strengthening those functions in the brain can help. If your child is struggling in school, consider the following functions that require brain networks and hubs working in sync to be successful:

- Ability to follow along in class (auditory processing, visual processing, attention, memory, fine motor)—a brilliant student who struggles to keep up with taking notes in class or writing down the correct directions to an assignment can still struggle if there is a disruption in any one of the skills contributing to this ability.
- Organization (memory, attention)—the act of forming or establishing something; cohesive notes from class to help study for a test, a clean bedroom with everything put in its proper place, or

the ability to utilize your backpack throughout the day to bring the necessary tools to class, including homework. A struggle with organization can result in a student who doesn't finish assignments on time or finishes the work but neglects to get it turned in on time. This student may excel when they do the work but have poor grades due to missed work. Test grades may be all over the place—if they study, they do well, but if they forget, or don't study effectively, it will be reflected in a low grade. This student may easily get overwhelmed and want to give up.

- Time management (memory, prioritization, attention)—the ability to use your time effectively or productively. This requires the ability to judge how much time it will take you to complete a task and to prioritize how you should be using your time. The student who struggles with time management is often running late and finds themselves stressed and irritable when running up against deadlines they aren't prepared to meet. Time management has been complicated with increased phone usage, as screen time has the power to hold our attention for long periods of time and distract us from what is going on around us.

Matthew was a classic example of a middle schooler struggling with organization and time management. He was a brilliant kid who tested well, but his inability to complete work and get it turned in hurt his grades and caused constant friction at home. When his mom reached out to me, she explained, "As the youngest of three boys, I know how much support I had to give the other two, and I've always known that Matthew needed more help and reminders, but I saw it getting *worse* over time, not better. Knowing what it has taken to keep him on track in middle school is scaring me for high school, and where he'll end up as an adult. I won't be here to hold his hand and nag him daily forever. His dad is convinced he's just lazy and doesn't care about school, but my gut tells me there is more to it—it's not just homework he forgets but soccer shoes for a soccer game, his lunch, you name it, he's just always in a state of chaos. We've tried everything from an organizational coach to medication, but we still feel stuck."

Going through an evaluation with Matthew, it quickly became clear that while he was thirteen years old, in several key developmental areas he was testing many years behind. Attention, memory, auditory processing, coordination, and functions that require multi-tasking of the brain tested especially low. So, while school had thirteen-year-old expectations for organization and follow-through, he had abilities more on par with an eight-year-old. Think how different your expectations are for a third grader versus an eighth grader. No wonder home and school environments were overwhelming and challenging.

I explained to Matthew's mom that after Matthew worked to mature and improve many brain functions, she could re-address the same organizational strategies the coach taught them—but she would be teaching a thirteen-year-old brain organizational strategies, which would be far more successful than trying to implement strategies with a third grader.

Neuroplasticity means the brain can change—and this contributes to our learning at all stages in life. But there is a sweet spot when these changes in the brain occur most efficiently. If something is too *hard*, we shut down and stop paying attention. If something is too *easy*, we can zone out and still do the work or complete the task. Like in the story "Goldilocks and the Three Bears," the conditions need to be just right.

Think of this sweet spot as the challenge point. It's the point in learning where you need to pay attention to think and make connections, and— voilà!—the brain will learn something new.

If your child has fallen behind or is really struggling in a class, it's possible that the material has gotten *too* challenging, and they've shut down or tuned out in this area. This is the time when spending more time reviewing content can be really helpful. You can't solve for *x* in algebra if you're still mastering basics like long division.

It's also important to get kids both aware of and comfortable with their challenge point. This can help them identify when things have gotten too hard, or why they aren't engaged. Teaching kids to work through this will help them later in life—as work and life in general will often throw you curveballs of new and difficult tasks. Getting used to being uncomfortable when something gets hard and working through it to the other side results in feelings of accomplishment, releases dopamine, and shows kids they're capable.

We faced a mounting challenge point in sixth grade with our son Drew in math that we hadn't seen coming, but in the end we realized how important it was to work through it. Math had always come easily for Drew. He was working a grade level ahead and independently, and we never checked his homework or helped him review concepts until we got an email from his teacher. Drew's grades in math were starting to drop from a combination of missing assignments and lower test scores. Thinking the issue was organization, I started checking his completion of assignments, but still not the work itself. The grades kept dropping and Drew started to talk about how much he hated this teacher and math itself.

I finally started to sit down with him while he did his assignments and realized there were several concepts he was missing: fractions and all the ways you manipulate them for multiplying and dividing. Working with him on this wasn't pretty—my calm, chill kid snapped a pencil in half, slammed his book shut, walked away, got angry—all the things you can imagine from a frustrated middle schooler. Math got hard, he didn't get it, and he wouldn't listen to help and guidance, so it wasn't getting any better.

The next email I got from the teacher suggested that he drop down a math level since he was struggling. This meant he would be repeating that entire year of math. This didn't make sense to me since the struggle was recent, not ongoing.

Watching Drew struggle with math revealed to me that he didn't handle an academic challenge well. At all. This hadn't happened before—it had been easy up until this point. He didn't need an entire year of review, he needed to learn how to dig in and do the work to push through. Luckily the email from the teacher about dropping down a level caught Drew's attention and pushed him to work harder. We sat down and planned to spend time together each night after dinner reviewing his work. We also agreed that if he started to act up, I was out of there. I was happy to help, but only if he was willing to try too.

I emailed the teacher to share my thoughts on Drew's need to learn to do the work when it gets hard and our plan for support. Luckily this did the trick, and Drew was able to quickly catch up (which was good, since I am not a good math teacher/helper). Not only did Drew need to learn more about fractions, he needed to learn how to study, review, and ask for help. I saw that Drew needed *more* hard in his life—not less.

The middle school and high school years are incredible for experiential learning, learning that takes place outside the classroom, involves all of the senses, and captures engagement.

Providing kids with the opportunity to expand their horizons and push boundaries will not only create lasting memories but also increase and expand their awareness of the world and just might enhance traits like empathy and understanding as well as confidence in themselves.

Thinking back on my own teenage years, so many of my vivid memories that sparked interest, fueled awareness, and even taught me life skills took place outside of school. My parents are big believers in providing kids a wide array of exposure and experiences, and for that I am grateful and hope to do the same for my kids.

One of my early memories of experiential learning was a summer science program at the local university that I did while in elementary school. It was in these classes that I first looked at a drop of lake water under a microscope to see all the living things in it, and then dissected a pig's eyeball. These classes sparked an early interest in science and anatomy—unlike my school science class, which to me felt boring.

In middle school, through our church youth group, I attended a day-long program where we were given a tour of downtown Minneapolis by a homeless person. They shared what their day looked like, the walk from the homeless shelter to the soup kitchen, and where they would go to sleep at night if the shelter was full. Walking the same Minneapolis skyway system my family would take to go to the Macy's Christmas display, but with a homeless person instead, showed me just how naive and unaware I was of the world beyond my bubble.

In high school my powerful experiential learning experience was getting to participate in the Appalachia Service Project, the same project that Noah would participate in years later. Not only did this bring me outside my suburban life in Minnesota, but these trips introduced me to roofing work; how to use a hammer, nail, and saw; minor plumbing repairs; and more. I learned to build something, to know that satisfaction and that feeling of accomplishment. Spending time with kids both older and younger from our group, getting to know the families whose homes we were helping to repair, taking cold showers, and sleeping on a cot in a hot gym at night increased my skills, confidence, and awareness of the world around me.

These experiences were not expensive in cost but were valuable in their lessons. The pandemic put us all on lockdown and changed the way we interacted for a time—minimizing the opportunities for experiential learning. Now we can re-emphasize these experiences for our kids by remembering that learning is more than what happens in school. There is tremendous value in finding ways to expand the horizons and experiences for our kids, helping to shape and inform their worldview to create better citizens for our communities.

Learning Development Activities for Middle School and High School Students

- Brainstorm together with your teen ideas for experiential learning—taking a class, signing up for a workshop, and volunteering are all great ways to learn outside the classroom
- Encourage your kids to do something hard and push through it
    - Not a runner? Have them sign up for a short race and make it happen. Read a book that intimidates them—in size or topic. Do these things together with your teen to challenge yourself as well, and provide support and accountability
    - Encourage your kids to do a crossword puzzle, sudoku, or jigsaw puzzle
    - Have them learn something new that interests them—how to play the drums or guitar, how to bake an amazing dessert, anything new, different, and challenging
- Encourage the use of a day planner
    - Work with your child to set a goal and use the planner to map out the steps and timeline to achieve the goal

o Show your teen how to map out time blocking and then hold themselves accountable to that time. If they gave themselves one hour for homework and thirty minutes for social media after—did they stick to the plan? Or did they cheat and glance at their phone when they got stuck on their homework?

• Are they struggling in a class or with a topic? Help them find ways to engage their senses while studying.

  o Encourage handwritten notes (not just rereading, typing, or circling information with a stylus on a tablet or chromebook)
  o Make flash cards using different color cards or pens to categorize the information
  o Add a physical movement to help remember specific details
  o Diffuse essential oils while studying
  o Exercise to re-engage the brain when feeling stuck
  o Draw out what they are learning. For example, in biology, draw out the steps of mitosis, or draw a flower and label the parts.
  o Use their phone to record themselves reading their notes out loud, then listen to this recording as a way to study.
  o Use mental imagery to visualize what they are reading or hearing to enhance memory.

• How to increase excitement around learning through leveraging the brain and the neurotransmitter dopamine:

  o Add novelty
  o Correlate what they're learning to something that matters/ motivates them; make it personal
  o Set a goal with an action plan of achieving it
  o Push past a challenge point for an achievement—whether they are completing a math homework assignment so that they feel confident in their work or building something for their science project, big or small, it will still feel rewarding

Signs That Indicate Improvement

The brain loves to learn, especially if it is studying an interesting topic. Watch for that joy or excitement that comes when the concept your child is working to master "clicks" for them. Even when hard, there is a sense of accomplishment when they finally get it. As the fundamental tools for learning start to improve, you will notice things clicking and sticking sooner with your child—there will be less repetition of the same information and an ability to recall it the next day rather than having to start over from scratch, and making connections and applying the information learned. Watch for your child to do the work more independently once they grasp the topic— whether they are learning colors, to read, or a concept, you will notice them demonstrating their newfound ability willingly. You will see fewer negative behaviors and less of the negative self-talk when it comes time to do work. And maybe, just maybe, they will start to actually enjoy elements of school and learning.

7
····

UNDERSTANDING UPSETS AND HOW TO MOVE PAST THE MOMENT

Upsets happen. It's a fact of life. The question becomes: Are the frequency and duration of behaviors on track with development? **When development is immature, a child (or adult) will have less of an ability to control their reactions and behaviors. There will be a lower threshold for what they are able to tolerate before the upset is triggered, and the upsets will tend to be bigger and last longer.** In this chapter we will discuss developmentally appropriate expectations for facing life's challenging moments, how to set appropriate expectations, and how to provide guidance and support to help your child move beyond the upset.

Note to Parents

If you've ever wondered if other parents face the epic meltdowns you experience or feel like you are walking on eggshells to brace for the next major upset, this chapter is for you.

Outbursts that seem longer, larger, or more frequent than those of other kids the same age may be a sign of immaturity in elements of development leading to control. (This does not mean that upsets shouldn't happen; they can and will for the rest of your life. The key is the ability to face life's challenges in an appropriate way for your child's age and stage of development.)

We've all been there. The screaming toddler under your arm while you're trying to push a cart through Target and not sweat through your shirt. The young child whose frustration builds to the point of lashing out physically. The ten-year-old shouting and arguing. The middle schooler giving you the stink eye, storming away, and slamming the door. The high schooler shutting down and retreating to their room. Indefinitely.

When moments like these occur, stress levels go through the roof, and constructive conversation goes out the window. The result can be anger, frustration, and even shame on the part of both the child and the parent. Understanding what triggers these moments and how the brain reacts will help you understand if your child is reacting in a way that is considered on track for their age. From there, you can implement strategies to help minimize or avoid these moments in the future.

Pandemic Lessons

The research is out, and the results are clear. Two-plus years of altered schooling and interactions left kids behind in social and emotional development. It's showing in classroom behaviors, with many schools reporting increases in disruptive behaviors, and at home as well.[1]

Our ability to identify what we are feeling and to communicate that information is directly tied to our development, which in turn affects our behaviors. Controlling our actions and reactions is also tied to development. The more mature we are in our development, the more able we are to dampen our impulses and *not* say out loud what we are thinking and *not* lash out when it isn't acceptable. The younger a child is developmentally, the less able they are to control their actions and reactions.

The reduction in face-to-face social interactions, reduced sensory exposure, less time on the playground navigating relationships and upsets, and more time at home with parents navigating challenges for their kids have all contributed to gaps in this area for many kids.

Add stress, change, or fatigue to the scenario and it's like pouring gas on a fire—the fire just gets bigger. Life is full of stress and change, so strengthening the networks in the brain that help our self-awareness, self-regulation, and *control* is necessary to support more age-appropriate behaviors in times of upset.

Science Alert

When we are relaxed, focused, and happy, our brain is easily able to utilize the networks that allow us to plan, think, communicate, and regulate our behaviors. But when an upset happens, this all changes. The levels of frustration slowly build until the breaking point. We all have one, and not only does it vary from person to person but it also can vary within the same person from day to day.

When it comes to upsets, I have a mental image: a person teetering on the edge of a cliff, trying not to fall. We all have a cliff; the question is, how far from the edge are you or your child on any given day?

Tipping over the cliff's edge is when your body shifts into "fight, flight, or freeze" mode. This nervous system response is a survival mechanism that prepares the body to fight or get away from danger. It puts your brain and body on high alert, shifting blood and energy to the body to prepare for protection and escape if necessary. Activity in the brain shifts from environmental focus to high alert as it takes in as much information as possible so you can react quickly. In these moments the brain is not thinking about long-term consequences or planning for the future but is focused on reacting to the perceived situation in that very moment.

The balance or calming mechanism to your fight or flight response is provided by the parasympathetic nervous system, mainly the vagal nerve. The more strongly engaged the vagal nerve is, the more you remain calm and relaxed, and the faster you can return to a state of calm as needed. This is not a single nerve but a bundle of approximately one million nerves that work cohesively as a system to maintain and restore calm in the brain and body, controlling heart rate, breathing, pupil dilation, and more.[2] The vast bundle of the vagal system is why, when you are really upset, startled, or stressed, a lot changes simultaneously. When vagal activation is *decreased,* the result is an *increase* of symptoms. Think of this like taking your foot off the brake— becoming upset or agitated removes the brake on the vagal nerve keeping your system calm. You may become flushed, agitated, experience increased respiration and hypersensitivity to sensory stimuli, or even develop an upset tummy (if you've ever experienced diarrhea at a time of stress, it is related to this system). Once the vagal system is deactivated (foot off the brake), it takes energy and activation *away* from higher-level pathways in your brain that would allow you to control your thoughts and actions and plan ahead. Instead, the energy is shifted to heighten sensory intake, increase reaction speed, and support muscles to run away from danger. Brain imaging during times of upset demonstrates increased activation in the amygdala, the emotional center of the brain, and decreased activity in the frontal cortex, the region of the brain that contributes to attention and impulse control.[3] This is why when you are *really* upset you are more likely to say and do things you ordinarily would not say or do. The brain at this point is functioning in the here and now—very reactively. Thinking through consequences, rewards, or reasoning becomes extremely difficult.

Understanding aspects of development that contribute to the maturation of these reactions and responses is what can point parents in a positive direction to support their children in times of frustration and upsets. **Research published in the journal** *Science* **examined how early life input impacts how the brain handles stress, reward, and fear. A key finding was that the maturation of sensory circuits influences emotional circuit maturation.**[4] A child's overall development will impact how well they tolerate and respond to upsets in life.

The goal of this chapter is to increase your understanding of what you can do to move your child further away from the edge of the cliff (strengthen the brake to provide more control and a faster return to a state of calm)—as well as handle the moments when your child has fallen off the edge.

Infants and Toddlers

Upsets in the infant years are more about communicating needs. When a baby is overly tired, hungry, or uncomfortable, crying is the only means they have to capture your attention so that you can provide whatever support is needed in that moment.

In the first few months with a newborn, it can feel like every day is different, but eventually you should start to see a general pattern emerge of times of sleep and wakeful engagement. Keep in mind that just when you think a routine has been established, teething, illness, and even bursts of development can derail the routine temporarily. The general trend, however, should be moving toward a pattern of sleeping and wakeful engagement.

As babies develop and become more engaged and more mobile, upsets are still a form of communication but also become a way to express frustration. They want a toy they can see but can't get to, or want to do something on their own but lack the coordination to make it happen. Remember that upsets are a normal part of the human experience; they simply present differently at differing ages and stages in life. Knowing what to watch for through these early years can provide both peace of mind and guidance to support your child if their reactions present as immature for their age. .

Upset Management Milestones for Infants and Toddlers (Understanding Age-Appropriate Behaviors and Reactions)

Up to three months:[5]
- Able to be calmed with rocking, touching, and gentle sounds

Up to twelve months:[6]
- Asocial, develops approach (positive behaviors such as smiling, eye contact, and cooing) and avoidance (negative behaviors such as turning the head, closing eyes, or crying) behaviors

One to two years:[7]
- May become angry if activities are interrupted
- Shows anger through aggressive behavior; may hit, bite, or fight over a toy
- Seeks comfort from caregivers—safe-base exploration (wandering only a few feet away, then returning to their caregiver, or staying within sight of the parent or caregiver)

Two to three years:[8]
- Screams, throws temper tantrums for little cause
- Is emotionally attached to toys or objects for security

Three to four years:[9]
- Demonstrates inconsistent behaviors
- Has no sense of privacy
- Is beginning to learn to take responsibility

Four to five years:[10]
- Exhibits increased frustration tolerance

- May show increased aggressive behavior
- Self-esteem reflects opinions of significant others
- Bosses and criticizes others
- Displays concern and sympathy

While parents are very familiar with the reality of the "terrible twos," they aren't always familiar with which aspects of upsets and meltdowns are age-appropriate for this age and stage, and when they are a sign of concern. Dr. Jay Hoecker of the Mayo Clinic describes this stage as one that includes "rapid shifts in mood and behaviors," and he acknowledges "the difficulty of dealing with them." He explains that at this age kids go through major motor, intellectual, social, and emotional changes and can typically understand much more language than they are able to speak.[11]

A 2003 study published in the *Journal of Developmental and Behavioral Pediatrics* determined that 75% of tantrums in kids ages eighteen to sixty months last five minutes or less and can also include physical reactions such as crying, hitting, kicking, biting, and throwing things.[12] So, while a toddler lashing out is stressful, it is an expected reaction to frustration at this age.

The expectation is that as the child continues to develop and mature, tantrums will become less frequent and less intense. According to Healthline, tantrums that fall outside age expectations could be indicative of other concerns. For ages three to six, things to watch out for include:[13]

- Tantrums lasting longer than twenty-five minutes
- Physically lashing out at a caregiver more than 50% of the time— hitting, kicking, biting
- Hurting self
- An inability for the child to eventually calm themselves
- Frequency of ten to twenty times per day

When kids are experiencing the symptoms listed above, it is an indicator that their fight or flight system is being triggered too easily, too often. They may also have a harder time transitioning out of fight or flight back into a relaxed, calm state. This is hard on everyone involved—the child who is in a state of extreme distress and the parent trying to manage the moment.

Our sensory processing can have a huge influence over our level of comfort in the environment and our tolerance for what is happening around us. Think of the last time you felt overwhelmed and stressed and lost your temper. For me, a combination of high stress related to work, a house that's a mess, dogs that are playing loudly, and kids who are not listening will likely make me feel overwhelmed and out of control, and that feels terrible. But I can verbalize my thoughts and reactions (and do so loudly).

Stress pushes us closer to the cliff's edge; adding a sensory load on top of that can simply be too much, pushing you over the edge.

The experience is similar for a child. Maybe normally they can handle the noise of a show in the background or the feel of a hot summer day, but add stress or uncertainty to the scenario and they're more likely to melt down. That sensory input on top of stress can be what pushes them over the edge.

Knowing how sensory stimulation can add to feelings of stress, uncertainty, overwhelm, and fatigue gives you a direction to go when you sense a meltdown approaching. Adjust the sensory input and do it fast.

Less is more at this point. Less noise, less visual input, less chaos. Removing a child from a busy environment, finding somewhere quiet and calm, then taking a moment to gently hold your child or place a reassuring hand on their head or back can help to avoid an oncoming upset.

If you're at a restaurant, go outside. At the park, go find some shade under a tree. At home, change rooms. In the car, turn off the radio and ask others to be quiet. In a line at Disney, sit down and create a quiet space on your lap with your child facing you to block whatever stimuli you can. At an indoor bounce park birthday party—get away as fast as you can (after two kids and dozens of birthday parties over the years, I can live a very fulfilled life never going to one of these places again).

While "less is more" is a helpful approach for everyone, at any age, it becomes even more necessary for a child who is dysregulated in their sensory processing. For that child, also address the upset by minimizing stimulation; then, when your child is rested, fed, and happy, work to provide as much physical activity and sensory stimuli as you can in small doses to exercise and use those pathways in the brain (refer back to chapter 2).

This advice doesn't apply just to our toddlers but to our older kids, spouse, and us as well. Picture family Thanksgiving. People and kids everywhere, the noise, the chaos. If you find yourself—or notice one of your kids—becoming irritable, take a break. Go for a walk. Even a few minutes of calm and quiet can help you move away from that cliff's edge so when the person next to you at the table brings up politics you can grin and bear it.

During an upset think "less is more" again, but for your *words* in addition to the sensory stimuli. Using fewer words is key, including not threatening a punishment or offering a reward. Now is not the time to have a discussion. Get through the moment, and then discuss after everyone has calmed back down.

When the brain hits that point of upset, activity shifts from thinking, planning, using logic, and problem solving to lower brain functions that support survival in that moment. The brain has a harder time processing information in this state. Your child simply will not hear and process what you are saying, so stop wasting your breath. Too many words will escalate, not calm, the situation.

In this moment as a parent, we need to do the opposite of what we are inclined to do. If a child is crying or upset, a parent will often talk louder or shout to get their attention or be heard over the noise of the child. This is more sensory input, not less, and aggressive tones, noises, words, or body language can be scary and intimidating for a child—pushing them further down the path of fight or flight rather than creating space for calm.

If you need to talk to your child, try to come *under* them, not *over* them with noise. Speak in a calm, quiet, soothing tone. Even whispering is different and can grab your child's attention. They may even quiet down for a moment to hear what you're saying (or maybe not). Stay quiet, calm, and patient. The outburst most likely won't get resolved in a minute or two at this point and that unrealistic expectation won't be helpful.

To increase the likelihood that your child will both hear and process what you're saying, use few words, with big spaces in between to allow more time for them to process what you are saying.

What you shouldn't say in this moment: "Stop! It isn't okay to hit someone, you need to learn to keep your hands to yourself. How would you like it if someone hit you? Stop crying now or we'll leave. You don't want to leave now, do you?" What will your child grasp from all of that? More noise bombarding their senses.

Try this instead: "Stop." Then give them a safe and quiet place and time to calm down.

Trying to motivate, rationalize, or discuss anything in this moment simply won't be effective. Instead, give your child time. When a person reaches the state of fight or flight, hormones are released in the body and stay active for several minutes. During this time, the emotional center of the brain will be the dominant controller. Once the body begins to calm down, the crying subsides, breathing slows, and the heart rate returns to normal. These are signs that the body is beginning to come out of the state of upset. This can take anywhere from twenty to forty minutes and may vary by person and intensity of the incident.

Once your child is quiet, calm, and relaxed, it is time to discuss what happened—at an age-appropriate level. Acknowledge their feelings. Everyone gets upset, and it is okay to feel angry (sad, hurt, scared—whatever is appropriate for the incident). "I know you're mad. It's okay to be mad. What isn't okay is hitting. Next time you are mad tell your friend why you are mad, and if they don't listen, then walk away."

Still, try to have this conversation with fewer words. Keep it simple and direct. In addressing an upset, I recommend focusing on three things—first, acknowledge how your child feels; even if you don't agree, it is real to them. Next, let them know you feel that way sometimes too; everyone does, it's okay. Then tell them an appropriate way to express themselves if they are mad, hurt, or scared.

It isn't realistic or even okay to *not* allow your kids to get angry or frustrated; we can't yell at them every time they get mad. Instead, we need to coach them in acceptable ways to handle the upset.

A good coach corrects in a way that sets an athlete up for success the next time the ball comes to them—do the same in your parenting.

I learned the art of patience with a toddler's tantrum because of babysitting my little sister Colleen. As the oldest of three girls, there were times when I was left in charge. I did not like this. At all. Colleen was (is) stubborn. I mean really stubborn. When she didn't get what she wanted, she could throw a fit like no other. She would spread her feet, stare you down, jut out her jaw, and let loose until she turned red and then purple in the face. With her flaming red curls and purple face of rage, she looked like she was going to explode. There was zero reasoning, bribing, or cajoling that would get her to stop once she started.

My mom taught me to walk away in this moment rather than try to interact with her. Not completely walk away, but go grab a kid's book, sit down, and start reading, just loud enough so Colleen could hear (between her screams when she needed to take a breath), but not so loud that you were shouting over her noise. Eventually, while taking a breath between bouts of her fit, she would hear a glimmer of the story and slowly start to quiet down to listen. (Even that young, she was so stubborn she would not climb into your lap to see the book, no matter how much she wanted to, but she would eventually quiet down and come close enough to see.) This would sometimes take reading more than one book, or the same book over and over, but each time she would eventually calm, and then it was like the tantrum never happened, except for evidence in her red, splotchy face and my level of stress.

I'm happy to report that she grew up to be a lovely adult and one of my favorite human beings. She also now has a daughter of her own (sweet justice). And as much as those moments stressed me out, they prepared me for babysitting and parenting in ways I couldn't appreciate back then.

When your child has tipped over the edge into a state of upset, it is not the time for rewards and motivation; but behavioral redirection can be beneficial in the time leading up to the upset and may help you navigate away from the cliff's edge.

When it comes to managing behaviors for little ones, think instant gratification. The younger the child is developmentally, the more immediate the reward or consequence needs to be for them to begin to connect the behavior with the outcome.

A young child has a very short attention span (think seconds, not several minutes or hours), they don't yet have a concept of time, and they are only beginning to learn the concept of cause and effect through play and trial and error. If I throw my bottle, you'll pick it up. This is a fun game, and it gets your attention.

Offering a reward that will come long after their attention span has run out is *not* the most effective strategy. "If you're good we'll go get ice cream after dinner!" By the time you go get the ice cream, your child will have forgotten why you're getting ice cream in the first place. If you want to use ice cream as the motivator, show your toddler the ice cream that's in your freezer and say, "You can have it when you're done."

Due to the naturally short attention span of toddlers, distraction can actually be an effective strategy to avoid an upset. Work to actively engage them in something other than what upset them in the first place. Sing, dance, clap. Turn out the lights. Anything to capture their attention and shift it from what frustrated or upset them to something else, to shift the focus of their mood and emotions.

If you see your child starting to get upset because the dog took their toy and ran away, simply grabbing another shiny toy and making it dance to capture your child's attention can be highly effective. The toddler's brain can only engage in one thing at a time and has an attention span of seconds to only a few minutes. Remember, mood and emotions shift quickly at this age; use this to your advantage.

The bottom line at this age is, the more instant and tangible the thing is you're using to redirect or motivate, the more helpful it will be. Using something they can see or touch can help to make it more real and motivating. Think stickers you keep in your purse, or a book or game you can read or play immediately.

We all have our own currency—the thing that motivates us. The trick is finding your child's currency. Potty training my son, Drew, showed us that at two years old his currency was Band-Aids. He had colorful Band-Aids up and down both legs because it was the one thing that motivated him to go sit on the potty chair. He looked ridiculous, but we didn't care since it did the trick. Books, games, treats, even stickers didn't work, but break out a Band-Aid and he was game (I still don't understand why a Band-Aid was okay and a sticker wasn't, but who am I to argue with a toddler?).

Next time your toddler is having a tantrum, reduce sensory stimuli in the moment, use fewer words, and distract them. These strategies, along with some patience, will help you both survive the incident with a little more ease. Then, in times of calm, continue to exercise and build their brain to increase their ability to regulate and control their reactions so you are faced with fewer tantrums going forward.

Upset Management Activities for Infants and Toddlers

- Use a day planner or journal to track your child's tantrum trends; knowing how frequently they occur and how long they last can help you understand if what you are experiencing is expected for their age or a red flag for concern. This can also help you spot trends to help you understand and manage the moments and will help you see if over time the upsets are getting better (which they should with age and development) or worse.
- Track what you notice in your child's behavior prior to a meltdown to help you spot the clues sooner to help navigate away from an upset in the future. Do they become hyper, quiet, or whiny? Do they become red and sweaty? Are there certain sensory stimuli that can push them over the edge: heat, loud noises?
- Ideas for instant gratification to motivate or redirect a behavior: playing with the family pet, giving stickers, finding a favorite toy, driving a toy truck across the floor, reading a book, playing a game, singing a song, doing a dance, coloring, going outside, changing the environment within the house, popping bubbles, changing the lighting in the room (turning a light off or on), drawing with sidewalk chalk, telling a story.
- Ways to change sensory stimulation:
  - Sight: Create calm visual input. Minimal or soft lighting is the goal. Turn off the television, close the curtains, or turn off the

overhead light. Pitch black may feel frightening; instead, turn on a lamp for softer lighting.

o Sound: Go under, not over, your child's voice; catch their attention by changing what you are doing. Whisper. Wait until they stop, then speak softly, calmly, quietly. Use as few words as possible until they are calm. Remove any additional possible auditory input such as television, music, siblings, or pets.

o Touch: Human contact has been shown to be calming (but may not work for everyone). Something as simple as a hand on the back or arm lets your child know you are there with them even if they don't want to be held.

Elementary School Students

In the elementary years, kids typically have a greater complexity of coordination, which allows them to accomplish more tasks on their own and to communicate what they want and need more effectively. However, at this age they are still learning to identify and communicate their emotions and to regulate their reactions. They are learning what is and isn't socially acceptable, and their increased awareness of peers and the world around them contributes to this learning process. A heightened sense of rules and right versus wrong can lead to impassioned feelings and responses: "He cut in line, he can't do that!"

Upset Management Milestones for Elementary School Students (Understanding Age-Appropriate Behaviors and Reactions)

Six to seven years:[14]
- May sometimes have temper tantrums

Seven to eight years:[15]
- Draws moral distinctions based on internal judgment
- Is self-critical; may express lack of confidence

Eight to nine years:[16]
- Becomes impatient; finds waiting for special events torturous

- Is influenced by peer pressure
- Seeks immediate gratification

Nine years:[17]

- Can control anger most of the time
- Has more stable emotions than the previous year
- Mood swings still occur but not as frequently as before

Nine to ten years:[18]

- Complains about fairness
- Can express a wide range of emotions

Ten to eleven years:[19]

- Becomes increasingly self-conscious
- Succumbs to peer pressure more readily
- Tries to avoid looking childish

Eleven to twelve years:[20]

- May be a repeat of the "terrible twos"
- Has little impulse control
- Is easily frustrated
- May feel out of control
- Can adapt behaviors to fit situations

As kids continue to develop and mature, how they act during times of upset will evolve to become quieter and more personal. In the elementary years, upsets will shift from loud wailing and crying to finding personal space and quiet to experience their strong emotions. Through these years kids become much more self-aware and aware of how others act and react around them in the classroom and on the playground. This awareness—if present and age appropriate—helps to shift their actions to be in line with those of their peers.

Understanding what is possible for your kids at this age, as well as what pushes them closer to and pulls them away from the cliff's edge, will help you navigate these years together.

Having realistic and developmentally appropriate expectations is key for parents to guide and support their kids through upsets. We discussed the importance of age-appropriate expectations for learning, but these expectations apply to behaviors and self-regulation as well. All too often I see parents with expectations for their child that simply aren't in line with reality. This sets both parent and child up for failure, disappointment, and frustration and can contribute to more meltdowns. Instead, focus on what your child *can do*, what they are capable of at this point in their life, and go from there.

This adjustment in expectations should apply to many areas: attention, impulse control, behaviors, discipline, chores around the house, following directions, and so on. If you're not sure what your kids are truly capable of doing, start by watching and taking notes.

Give your child a one-step direction. See if they can carry that out without additional prompts. If that is successful, next time try a two-step direction. Keep observing and building from there.

Maybe you'll find that when they're rested and calm, they can handle three steps, but when tired and cranky one step at a time is the max they can handle. This is typical; as adults we're the same way. Use that knowledge.

Usually, our support actions for our kids help them work toward greater independence—being able to get ready in the morning for school without us doing every step for them or being able to regulate their behavior when they're upset so they don't act out. But we aren't supporting independence by asking for more than they can do. So while it might be ideal to not have to remind them to hang up their wet towel and brush their teeth every night, you may need to until their development kicks in enough for them to do it (or choose to do it) on their own.

The goal here is not to let your child "get away" with more or refuse to hold them accountable for their actions. The goal is to meet your child where they currently are—then work to drive support and growth in these areas, so that over time you *can* have age-appropriate expectations for your child that they are able to meet. It feels so much better to meet or even exceed expectations than to fall short and disappoint those around you.

Think about how you would feel if your boss called you right now and said, "I need you to do [something you don't know how to do or aren't good at doing]. I need this done by the end of the day, it's important." What would this do to your stress levels? Your focus and motivation? Knowing you were asked to do something you're not capable of or not good at, and it needs to be done well and quickly? Yikes. No thanks. I'd be majorly stressed and super irritable.

Then the next day your boss calls to say, "I'm so disappointed in how you handled this project. I asked you to do X and you didn't do it." I would feel beyond awful. I'd be in a horrible mood, feel sick to my stomach, and probably have a hard time sleeping that night. The negative self-talk would kick in: "I can't do this, this is too hard. I'm out—I need to do something else."

Now think about how you'd feel if that same boss called to say, "You nailed it! Not only did you do exactly what I asked you to do, but you surpassed my expectations!" Woohoo! That phone call is one I'd be happy to answer any day. That one would motivate me to continue to work, and in fact I would probably work even harder to earn even more positive feedback.

A great leader understands your abilities—your strengths and weaknesses—and guides you on how to use those best. They still encourage you to do things that are hard, to help you grow and get even better.

Be honest with yourself about your child and their current abilities so that you can be that great leader to support them and help them grow. Meet them where they are currently and move forward together from there.

Giving your child the time and space to explore their abilities just might surprise you both. My sister Colleen learned this with her daughter, Anna, who loves *The Great British Baking Show*. There was a beautiful Christmas recipe on the show that Anna decided she was going to make. She was eight years old, and while she had often helped in the kitchen, this recipe was very involved. Kransekake, a traditional Scandinavian dessert, uses twelve individual ring pans and requires dough to be rolled out, then placed into the rings to bake. Next you stack the twelve rings, forming the shape of a Christmas tree. There is also frosting and glitter involved. Lots of glitter. It required a special set of pans and hours of work to bake, assemble, and decorate. My sister agreed to buy the pans, thinking it would be a good activity to do together over the holidays. But when the pans arrived, Anna went to work—on her own. The result was a gorgeous and delicious Scandinavian cake, a beyond proud eight-year-old, a trashed kitchen, and a new annual tradition. Giving Anna the space to read the directions, ask questions as needed, and do it on her own exercised her executive function pathways and built her joy and confidence in baking. She still is an incredible cook four years later, and my sister is happy to clean up the kitchen in exchange for her desserts and homemade sushi. Colleen never would have realized her daughter's talent and abilities had she not given her the space to try.

Trying new experiences with kids doesn't always go as well as baking did for Anna. A few months ago, I took Drew for a haircut, and the scene that unfolded in front of us was painful. While Drew and I were waiting for his turn, I visited with the parents sitting next to me. Both Mom and Dad were there, and the little girl, who was almost seven, was about to get her first haircut. Mom shared she had trimmed it at home from time to time, but this was her daughter's first time getting a professional haircut, which is why her hair was extremely long. When the mom and daughter walked away to look at something, the dad shared that his daughter screamed and cried when anyone tried to brush her hair but also didn't want anyone to cut it. But with long hair, the tangles just weren't manageable, so they wanted her to have a cute shorter haircut.

You could see the parents trying to build up her excitement, pointing out other kids sitting nicely and how great their hair looked when they were done. You could also see the fear and trepidation on the little girl's face; she was clinging to her mom, burying her face in her lap, and trying to change the subject from talking about haircuts.

The family had just come from a few hours of swimming at their neighborhood pool and were hoping to squeeze this in before grabbing a late lunch.

I'm sure by now you can imagine what I was thinking: *there's no way this is going to end well.* You have a tired, hungry child with sensory sensitivities who doesn't want a haircut. While kind and well-meaning, these lovely parents were doing nearly everything they could to ensure an epic meltdown was coming. For the sake of that sweet little girl, I wanted to be wrong, but unfortunately, I wasn't.

They called her name and she instantly started pulling her mom toward the door, not the chair. Both parents started talking to her over the stylist. Mom was bribing, "If you do this, we'll go out for ice cream with sprinkles after dinner!" Dad was alternating between threatening, "I'll take away your iPad if you don't cooperate!" and reasoning, "Let her cut your hair now and you won't have the tangles anymore and you can brush your own hair." The stylist was trying to distract her by asking which fun chair she wanted to sit in and if she had a favorite show or video game she wanted to play while getting her hair done.

This scenario was most likely going to be stressful no matter what; however, the parents were checking all the boxes to put her closer to the edge. Fatigue? Check, she had just been swimming for hours in the hot sun. Hungry? Check, they had skipped lunch and were going to eat later. Sensory stimuli, check, check, and check. A noisy salon with a toddler crying, video games playing, music blaring through the speakers, and three adults talking to her at once. I was on sensory overload as an adult sitting in this salon.

As the little girl's level of stress and upset escalated to a full meltdown, the parents upped their volume and what they were trying to discuss with her. They were trying to offer a reward—but delayed by hours, and they were trying to reason with her when she was in fight or flight.

The result was the three of them storming out without a haircut. The little girl was hysterical by this point, Dad was furious that they didn't see it through, and Mom looked near tears herself as she tried to hold and soothe her daughter.

With the eloquence of a twelve-year-old boy, Drew looked at me and said, "Well, that sucked."

"Yeah. It really did. And don't say suck."

My heart hurt for that family. With all good intentions, the parents unknowingly pushed the little girl closer to the edge of her cliff and she tipped over. That little girl was feeling horrible, and the parents were incredibly stressed out and frustrated with both each other and their daughter. And while it appears like a haircut will be challenging for this child for a while, there were so many things the parents could have done differently had they known.

To be clear, I am not judging these parents at all. I wanted to run out and shout, "Let me help you make a plan for next time!" They weren't bad parents, they just weren't well equipped for that moment.

We've all been there in one way or another, and it is much easier to see a situation clearly as an observer than as an active participant.

The example of the little girl's haircut-that-wasn't illustrates the things that push us closer to the edge. The list of activities in this section focuses on what you can do for your kids to *maximize* the buffer zone. The big-picture goal is to improve development and control in the brain through the developmental strategies outlined in this book. But there are day-to-day strategies that can be implemented to help minimize the upsets and maximize the good!

Upset Management Activities for Elementary School Students

While kids at this age can seem more independent and mature at times, there are other times when you are needed to step in to guide, direct, and co-regulate until they have the developmental ability to do this on their own. Here's a list of things to keep in mind to increase the buffer between your child and an upset, to minimize the need for help, support, and meltdowns:

- Rest—Do the new activity when your child is well rested, such as in late morning
- Fuel—Eat before activities, and make the food something with protein and healthy fats, not high in sugar, to provide sustained energy rather than a spike and a crash
- Sensory stimuli—Minimize the sensory experience so the brain doesn't get fatigued and overwhelmed. An example for the haircut scenario would be to find someone who can come to your home to cut your child's hair in their own calm, quiet, and familiar environment. This can help avoid the extra input of blow dryers, water running, and other people talking.
- Developmentally appropriate expectations—If your child is immature in their reaction to upsets, set your expectations for how you would manage a much younger child in this scenario. Plan to keep the potentially stressful activity short in duration, and describe to your child what will happen so they know what to expect. Reassure them that you will be there with them. Keep in mind that your calm presence can help co-regulate your child, even if they are older.

Co-regulate simply means to do something together; you are working with your child to help them return to a state of control and calm. Holding them on your lap or putting a soothing hand on their arm or back and saying calm words may provide a sense of comfort and safety. You can bring along a small toy or activity for distraction, such as stickers or coloring books, that can allow your child to focus on something they enjoy doing. Be sure to introduce this fun activity before they are upset and not during the upset.

- Less is more—Few words spoken quietly, rather than many words with reasoning and logic, will have an impact in this moment. "It's okay." Pause. "I'm here." Pause. "You got this." Keep this soothing support to one person speaking, and not multiple people trying to step in and help.

- Their pain or concern is real to them—Talk about what to expect and acknowledge how they feel about the activity or upcoming event. For the haircut example, the parent could have set the expectation by stating something along the lines of, "I know having your hair brushed is uncomfortable to you. It is time for you to get a haircut, so we need to do this, but we'll work together to do it as fast as we can so it is over quickly. If you need to take a break, let us know and we can do that, but we will finish." Then, during the haircut, still acknowledge how she feels: "I'm sorry you're scared [uncomfortable, angry, etc.], I'm here."

- Quiet recovery time once fight or flight has occurred—Once the upset escalates, find a calm, quiet environment and allow time for their system to reset, even if it takes twenty minutes or more. Then return to the activity when your child has calmed down and recovered—with distraction in hand.

- Exercise—Engaging in physical activity can help activate the RAS, the part of your nervous system that signals your brain to wake up and pay attention. (For a review of this information, re-read chapter 1, where we discuss core muscles.) If your child is becoming tired, sluggish, burned out, or irritable, that can be a good time to stop what you are doing and move. This can help prepare their brain to refocus to gain some additional minutes of productivity. When taking a movement break, do something that causes your child to go breathless (that moment when you need to pause to catch your breath). This activation is like exercise for the calming mechanisms in the brain (to learn more about the power of exercise, be sure to read chapter 8).

- Balance—Timing is everything. If you know a particular moment may trigger a meltdown, do something fun first. It doesn't have to be for long, just long enough to ensure a happy, positive frame of mind—but not long enough to get tired. If your child loves games, play a game of Spot It together prior to pulling out the math homework. Then tell them you can play again after the math is completed if they hang in there. This will start your child further away from the edge and give them a reward to look forward to.

- Confidence—Approaching anything in life with a positive attitude does make a difference. A research paper titled "The Neurobiology of Confidence" discusses confidence as a core cognitive process that helps to optimize behaviors, including learning and reasoning.[21] Confidence increases our mental and emotional well-being, supporting our actions and behaviors in a positive manner. Finding ways to build confidence in general can help the brain approach hard moments in more calm, positive, and focused ways, rather than in fight or flight mode. You can also build confidence in the areas that cause your child stress and trigger upsets. If your child hates math, and homework time is a nightmare, it can be helpful to go back to a topic they have already mastered to show them, "Hey! You've got this! Remember when this was so hard for you? You CAN do this! Now, let's practice this next topic until this one is easy too."

- Practice—You utilize a specific set of pathways in the brain each time you do something, whether it is practicing math facts, writing an essay, having a tough conversation with a friend, or improving in your sport. The more you practice, the easier it is to access those same pathways again. For me, doing something such as trying to assemble an Ikea bookshelf just may put me over the edge. To avoid a meltdown in the future, I should do more tasks that require reading every single detail, practice following step-by-step directions, and work on visual spatial memory by doing a large puzzle (absolute torture for me—I'm the cook who prefers to not follow a recipe and would rather clean the house than do a puzzle).

- Chunking—Don't expect your child to do too much all at once. Remember, it's not only okay but can be helpful to take breaks, ideally with physical activity to help reset the brain. Whether it's cleaning their room or doing homework, keep their window of attention in mind and be careful not to push too far past it.

Middle School and High School Students

In some ways, the teen years can feel like the toddler years all over again as our kids rush toward independence. They assert their thoughts, ideas, and opinions and want to do things their way and on their own. Their dependence at this age shifts from us to their peers as they work to find their community and build meaningful connections outside the home. While watching your child grow can be thrilling, it is also a time ripe with concern as our kids fly farther and farther from the protection of our home nest and venture out into the world on their own.

This age comes with a larger knowledge base of what they should do to take care of themselves, but knowing and doing are two separate considerations. To quote my husband, Doug, "First you need the neurology in order to apply the psychology." In other words, you need the developmental ability to apply what is needed in order to have success. You know you should take time to yourself to calm down when really angry, but the ability to control your action in that moment is dependent on your development to provide you with the necessary control.

Upset Management Milestones for Middle School
and High School Students (Understanding
Age-Appropriate Behaviors and Reactions)

Thirteen to fourteen years.[22]
- Can be inconsistent and unpredictable

- Can show extreme emotions
- Has inadequate coping skills

Fifteen to seventeen years:[23]

- Goes through less conflict with parents, shows more independence from parents
- Feels a lot of sadness, which can impact grades and choices regarding drug and alcohol use, sexual behaviors, and other activities

Life and parenting were already hard, and now we've added hormones?! Deep breaths. You've got this. It's true that upsets and anger change with time and hormones. As your child's brain and body begin to go through puberty, there is a new layer of complication. Add to that the pressures of school as they get older, a need for social acceptance, and the introduction of romantic interests, and as a parent you're facing a minefield of emotions that could go off at any moment. Co-regulation can be harder at this age as they more frequently spend time upset alone in their room, but it still is needed at times. At this age it can be in the form of gentle guidance. First, helping your teen build their awareness of how stress and frustration impact how they feel can help them navigate this time, as well as their future. Next, it's helpful to find ways for them to have a little control in some areas of life. Finally, learning how to recover from an upset when it happens can help get through challenging moments in life—while they are still working to build and strengthen the brain.

With added hormones come larger swings in mood and emotions, which can leave your teen feeling more out of control and reactive than ever. On top of the hormones, an increasing awareness of the world can contribute to feelings of anger. An injustice in the world, or how someone has been treated, can trigger anger, especially if something feels big or beyond their influence.

As a teenager I had an instance of extreme fright leading to extreme anger toward friends. I had a job working at a department store at the local mall, and I often worked the evening shift. This meant walking to my car in the dark and cold. I drove my mom's minivan to work, and since I had a bad habit of locking keys in the car, my dad had gotten me a magnetic key box. The problem was, my friends also knew about the key box (I'm sure you can guess where this story is headed). The two friends, who shall remain un-named, decided to visit me one night at work, but since they got there late, the stores were closed—and due to the bitter cold they decided the best idea was to take advantage of that key and wait *in* my car. While waiting they got the not-so-funny idea to crouch behind the seats and surprise me.

I hopped in the front seat of the minivan and as I started to put my keys in the ignition there was a loud "Boo!" from behind me. I started screaming and couldn't stop. My friends started laughing, and somewhere in the recess of my mind I knew I recognized those giggles, but not enough to stop the screaming. Eventually they crawled up front where I could see them, to try and reassure me I was safe. But it was too late for my nervous system. I was frozen in fight or flight mode—which is sometimes called fight, flight, or freeze for very good reason. Lucky for them I was frozen in fear, otherwise I would have used the Mace on my keychain. I couldn't even turn around to see who was there.

My screams subsided to shaking, then my emotions shifted over to anger. It took nearly thirty minutes before I was calm enough to drive home, before my nervous system could reset to be able to think and process informa-tion. While my calm returned, the resulting emotion was anger. I was *mad* that what they did stressed me out to the point of feeling so vulnerable and scared.

Our friendships did survive this incident, although clearly I still remem-ber it vividly. The prank did show me a real-life example of exactly how the nervous system reacts and recovers with fear and anger.

My reaction was completely normal and justifiable, but to make me feel a bit better I needed to do a few things to provide myself with a sense of control over my situation, and I needed time for my anger to subside. There was nothing that could be done to minimize my reaction to that startle expe-rience in my car, but I was able to make myself feel a bit better going forward by always checking the backseat of my car, never using a magnetic key box again, and carrying Mace in my hand, not just on my keychain.

Finding ways to help your teen develop a sense of *control,* even if small, over some aspects of life and *independence* in at least a few areas can create a sense of capability in self and calm.

This doesn't mean teens get to make *all* their own decisions; choose some areas where they can. Then, with success, you can start to expand that range of independence. This will look different for each child depending on their development and abilities.

A great but small place to start in the early tween years can be the grocery store. Sending your child into the store with money, a task, and a budget can be a great starting point. "Grab what you want the family to have for dinner tonight. Here's $30. Make sure there's a protein and a vegetable, please!" Not only are they practicing a life skill used daily (budgeting and grocery shopping), but they get to choose what they want to eat that night. If planning dinner is too overwhelming, start smaller—have them pick out a snack or beverage.

You may be asking yourself what grocery shopping has to do with meltdowns in teenagers. When the world is spinning around them and they're struggling, finding small things they can control can feel good and independent. Calming.

See the activities section for a list of ideas and ways to start to increase independence in your teens.

If you're noticing your teen tipping into anger, uncontrollable stress, or their fight, flight, or freeze mode too often, focusing on development and strengthening the pathways in the brain can help. Whether a history of developmental immaturity or trauma has set the stage for this hypersensitive trigger to extreme emotion, exercises and strengthening foundational development can help lead to a larger threshold of reaction. Go back to the basics to engage and improve how the brain takes in and responds to information and stimulation (refer to chapters 1, 2, and 3). Sensory stimulation, physical exercise, coordination, and timing are all categories that lead to improved processing of information, and improved control for how you respond to that information. At this age daily life doesn't involve play the way it did in younger years, which means it can be easy to skip this input to the brain.

Without intentional thought to stimulate the senses and muscles, movement can easily fall away and be replaced by sedentary activities. Don't forget how important movement and the senses are to orient and calm the brain and body. Find ways to play and move at all ages. Research shows that aerobics, yoga, and mindfulness can be great ways to engage the brain and body, positively impacting reasoning, memory, and self-control.[24] (See the activities list for additional ideas.)

Next, to help your teen improve their emotional regulation, exercise the pathways used in their executive functions. While many things fall into the category of executive functions, there are three overarching components that contribute directly to handling mood and frustrations. These main categories are inhibition, working memory, and cognitive flexibility.

Inhibition allows you to choose how you direct your attention and stops you from acting on impulse, which impacts behavior. Inhibition is your control of body and behaviors. A lack of inhibition will contribute to focused attention being directed in the wrong way, or in environmental attention allowing your thoughts to wander. When inhibition is low, you may have a hard time *stopping* an activity and transitioning to something else. Turning off the game to sit down for dinner or homework, for example.

Working memory refers to the information you keep active in your mind long enough to use or adapt and apply. Your working memory allows you to keep your task list active in your brain long enough to complete the list, even if it means doing the tasks out of order. It's hard to follow directions or complete a task if you can't remember what you are trying to do, or the steps you were asked to complete. Disruptions in working memory can leave you feeling lost, behind, and confused.

Cognitive flexibility is the ability to change directions or tasks—to adapt your plans or your day based on changing circumstances—without derailing your mood or energy. Your ability to shift from task to task and go with the flow is based on your level of cognitive flexibility. A recent study out of the University of North Carolina showed that kids with ADHD have a much harder time with this flexibility. Specifically, pathways involved with sensory, motor, and visual information are impacted.[25] The result is that more energy and effort need to go into anything requiring cognitive flexibility, which quickly drains resources. This becomes a negative spiral, where a tired brain has a harder time focusing and making good decisions. Your cognitive flexibility should improve over time with development. This flexibility can impact many areas, including how stressed you become with changes as well as planning, organization, and time management.

Remember, the more you use a pathway, the more efficient it will become. Doing activities to target the pathways involved in sensory, motor, visual, and executive functions can contribute to improvements in these areas, resulting in better outcomes that use less energy. (See the activities section for ways to exercise these functions.) Research indicates that executive function skills need to be repeated to be improved and must be progressively challenging.[26] As you improve, the challenge level needs to increase.

Upsets will happen at this age, it's a part of life. Work with your teen on building their interoception, their awareness of what they're feeling and when. It is okay and normal to feel all the emotions, it's how you handle those emotions that can take a lot of learning and growth. It's normal to feel stressed; now encourage them to dig deep to realize in themselves what escalates that stress and frustration. Disruptions with friends, upcoming tests, homework piling up? Pressure and expectations from parents? Siblings?

Identifying the stressors doesn't always mean they can be changed. But you can start by acknowledging what is contributing to the stress; this can lead to action plans to help mitigate the stress.

It's a matter of learning to stop and take your emotional temperature—how hot or cold are you running today? Then take a step back and consider why.

For years I've driven my kids to school early each morning. Most mornings I'm groggy but in a good mood, or at least as good as it gets that early. But then there are those mornings that I'm irritable and will snap more easily—at the kids for not putting away their breakfast mess, at Morgan for running late when getting ready, at anything and everything. The reality is each morning has its challenges, but I don't lose it each morning. As I'm driving along on those mornings when my mood is teetering on the edge of the cliff, I've gotten better at pulling back and looking at why. Have I been getting enough sleep? Am I stressed about something at work? Do I

have a headache, so the discomfort is lowering my threshold? Once I identify what is impacting my mood, I think about how I can impact it to shift
my thoughts and feelings. Fuel and exercise are often the two approaches
most readily available to help your child (or you) pivot a moment relatively
quickly. Remember, depleted resources and energy will result in increased
negativity. Stopping in that moment to take a few minutes to spike the heart
rate can impact mood and hormones quickly. Eating can provide fuel for
the brain that can impact a mood in as short a time as the twenty minutes
or so it takes for the body to begin to put those resources to work. Encourage your child to ask themselves, "Do I need to have a conversation to get
a lingering challenge off my mind?" If so, make a to-do list with a plan of
how to address what is contributing to feeling overwhelmed. Taking just five
minutes to write things down and map out a timeline can provide a sense of
increased calm.

Improving my own mindfulness, my self-awareness of feelings and actions, has helped me guide my kids through this same process. When Drew
is feeling stressed or upset, he gets incredibly negative. He hates everything,
and everything is useless. His stress or anger shuts him down. Guiding him
to proactively address this has helped—knowing there are times he will feel
stressed and anxious, like before a big test or game, allows me to help him
prep. "It's normal to feel negative when you're worried. How can I help you
today so you feel more prepared or equipped for what needs to happen and
are less stressed?"

The goal is not to solve all your child's challenges but to guide them
through navigating life's moments so that you can pull back, allowing them
the space to handle things on their own as they mature.

As hard as we try to avoid getting to that point of falling off the cliff's
edge, for our kids and ourselves, it still happens. When it does, knowing
what the brain needs to move through the moment and recover can help
minimize the fallout of the upset. Becoming fluid in implementing healthy
and appropriate ways of dealing with big feelings and emotions is a skill that
will help throughout life, not just those teenage years.

Let's review what we discussed earlier, since it applies to all ages in many
different scenarios. Once the fight or flight mode is activated in the brain,

it takes time to return to a state of calm. Learning to give yourself time and space is so important, as otherwise you might say and do things you wouldn't normally. Just like the toddler in the middle of a tantrum, once in this state, the brain loses the capability to use logic and reasoning and has less control. Allow your kids to press pause in this moment. As the parent, guide them through this until they can recognize the moment and make the choice to pause on their own. "You're upset right now. Let's set this conversation aside and finish talking in an hour, after you've calmed down and eaten." Acknowledge how they are feeling. Even if you don't agree, it is the state they are in—mad, stressed, scared, sad.

The brain will need at least twenty minutes of calm and quiet to begin to reset. Trying to push through the moment too soon will only escalate the situation again. Don't raise your voice, have an aggressive body posture, or get in their personal space. All these things will be perceived by a stressed-out brain as aggressive, which can escalate, not de-escalate, the fight or flight response. This is also not the time to talk—not about rewards or consequences, not about reasoning or logic. Just. Get. Through. It. Then, once everyone is calm and collected, you can discuss.

Everything we discussed earlier in this chapter for the infant/toddler brain applies to this age as well when the upset has peaked. The brain at this point needs calm, quiet, and soothing to return to feeling safe and in control once again.

To allow the calming mechanism to kick in faster, purposeful engagement of the vagal nerve—the longest nerve in our body—can help. Remember, this nerve impacts the heart, lungs, and your digestive system as well as muscles in your face, neck, and shoulders. Purposeful slow breathing, tensing and relaxing muscles through exercise or relaxation techniques, and eating (chewing and swallowing) all utilize this bundle of nerves.[27] See the activities section for more strategies.

The more mature the brain, the better equipped your kids are to handle upsets. The less mature, the more guidance and support your kids will need until they have the developmental capabilities to apply these strategies on their own. Don't forget that the strength and efficacy of brain networks is not directly related to age—so just because they're sixteen, twenty-six, or forty-six doesn't mean they'll automatically have the necessary higher brain networks needed to self-regulate.

Even though teenagers have glimmers of maturity, they still don't have the fully formed networks and pathways in their brain required for consistently good decision making, planning, and organization. Providing them structure and allowing them some space for their growing needs and desire for independence can be a delicate balance. They may not have the maturity to choose what they *need* over what they *want.*

Letting your middle schooler decide how late they'll stay up can be a major hazard for their ability to control and regulate their focus and emotions the next day. A tired brain just does not operate as well as a rested brain. At any age. And remember, they already have less development in the networks for executive functions, so adding fatigue will make everything harder.

Your priority for them and their priorities for themselves may not be the same. At this age, peer acceptance and a full social calendar begin to take on a greater role in their life, while you may be more focused on their emotional well-being and performance in school. Sit down and talk. Discuss with each other what is important to you and why, and then talk about ways to achieve both goals. For example, they can spend time with friends on the weekend if they consistently get work turned in and maintain certain grades in their classes that week.

Focusing on building the brain through sensory stimulation and physical engagement while increasing self-awareness will be a huge step toward improved awareness, control, and decision making!

Upset Management Activities for Middle School and High School Students

Start thinking and working proactively with your teen: "I know this is going to be a really busy week between school and sports—what do you think would be some good things to focus on this week to help? Lots of sleep, healthy breakfast, healthy snacks?" Think about ways to minimize stress: to-do lists, organization, help studying, and so on.

Other opportunities for a teen to build feelings of control and independence:

- Plan groceries and meals—breakfast, lunch, and snacks—for the week with a budget
- Be in charge of family dinner one night per week—choosing a recipe, getting the ingredients, and prepping the meal
- Order school supplies for the year—also with a budget and a list of what is needed, including the necessary shoes and clothing to start the year
- Shop for gifts for friends and family
- Select a project around the house and handle it from beginning to end: Organize the pantry, the linen closet, or their closet. Repaint the deck. Plant a garden. Mow and edge the yard. Bathe the dog.
- Get a job. Getting hired and trained, doing the work, and earning their own money is one of the biggest ways to build independence. Whether it's babysitting, mowing lawns in the neighborhood, or working at the local grocery store, having a schedule and responsibilities that they need to balance with school and socializing is something they will carry with them for life.
- Write it down. My dad taught us to make a list when my sisters and I were faced with a big decision or felt stressed. His favorite was the pros/cons list. I wanted to get another family dog and I was trying to convince him it was a good idea, so I made a pros and cons list for everything. Different breeds, sizes of dogs, should we even do it? While being asked to make a list as a child felt annoying in the moment, I still make those lists today, and it does help me think things through step-by-step to create a plan. I find lists especially helpful when things are weighing on my mind. I write down everything I need to do, then group the list in order of importance and due date. Then, I try to get the worst tasks out of the way first, to start to provide a sense of relief. And then I relish the sensation of checking something off the list.

- Utilize the power of exercise and movement to impact mood and as a positive strategy to help manage stress

Activities to help your teen find ways to "play" and move at all ages to engage the senses and the muscles:

- Explore nature—hike, bike, swim, run, walk nature trails or the dog
- Cook—find recipes online that look delicious or take a cooking class
- Make arts and crafts—find ideas on Pinterest
- Explore photography—experiment with your phone or with a traditional camera and lens; watch YouTube videos to learn how
- Take up videography—capture what you love through video
- Explore various physical activities and adventures—try frisbee golf, ultimate frisbee, rock climbing, kayaking, paddleboarding, mountain biking, bowling, goat yoga, or Pilates; join a ninja warrior gym or visit a trampoline park or a skate park
- Enjoy theater—watch or participate. Act, dance, sing, try improv comedy

Activities to practice executive function skills: reasoning, memory, self-control, organization, planning, time management, follow-through (but remember that practice alone won't get you there—build the brain and then exercise the pathways through practice):

- Encourage your student to use a daily planner. Create lists of what needs to be done and plan out their days in time blocks to get things completed on time. Each time they do this activity, they are engaging the pathways needed to plan and execute.
- If going on a trip, ask your teen to help you plan the route, including where you'll stop for gas and the best rest stops along the way. Any fun sights worth stopping to check out en route? Unique or quirky restaurants to explore?

- Make impulse control practice a game. Choose a word and for a dinner or a day you can't use the word. It can be any word you use often—like *you* or *the*. As you're talking, can you be aware enough to stop yourself from saying the word out loud?
- Adjust your timing—changing your natural timing requires self-awareness and control. When you go for a walk or run, do it at a different pace. Both faster and slower are hard, but for different reasons.
- Set a goal of not using the snooze button on your alarm—it takes great self-control to get up and moving the first time.
- Activities to engage the vagus nerve for a calming effect:
  - Practice deep belly breathing
  - Purse lips to blow air out (the lips contain parasympathetic nerve fibers)
  - Chew and swallow
  - Gargle
  - Give yourself a facial massage, rubbing eyes, lips, cheeks
  - Tense and relax muscles
  - Exercise
  - Practice gratitude (keep a journal or think about what you are thankful for)
  - Meditate
  - Provide a gentle touch, such as a hug or a light back rub or a comforting hand on their arm, to let them know you are there
  - Put something cold on the back of the neck—ice or a cold, wet towel

Signs to recognize a potential meltdown:

- Fatigue
- Hunger
- A shift or change in energy—becoming hyper or sluggish
- Becoming flushed in the face or having clammy hands

- Struggling to make a decision and becoming irritable if pushed to decide
- Losing attention and focus, even if doing something they typically enjoy
- Prolonged time in a highly stimulating sensory environment (the mall, a busy park or pool)

Signs That Indicate Improvement

As your child matures, the upsets will become less frequent, less intense, shorter in duration, and, over time, more private. You'll notice an increase in communication—which may look like talking back: "Mom, I *am* cleaning my room right now." Allow for communication to happen around upsets—give your child the opportunity to express their frustrations and why they feel that way. This is a necessary and helpful skill throughout life. You can still set boundaries: "It's okay to tell me you're mad and why, but not okay to use rude words when you do."

As development progresses, you'll see an increase in self-awareness of what triggers an upset and how to manage actions and words in the moment. Remember, this doesn't mean your toddler or teen will no longer fall off the cliff's edge; it means they'll manage it better when it happens.

8

. . . .

ANXIETY AND THE BRAIN

Note to Parents

When it comes to anxiety, I've always wanted to better understand why one person perceives an event as stressful while another does not. I saw this stark difference in reactions to stress when I took a group of kids to an indoor water park. Three nine-year-old girls on one giant waterslide. Two had the time of their lives. One had a panic attack. Why? Her panic attack was not due to a lack of coping strategies but to a difference in how her brain processed and reacted to the ride. Everyone experienced the same event and adrenaline rush, but for one brain it was just too much. While this was simply heartbreaking for me to watch, it spurred awareness of anxiety and my interest in learning how to impact the brain to lessen this response.

Racing heart, sweaty palms, upset stomach, feelings of dread or avoidance: Symptoms of anxiety can happen to any of us, at any age. While there are elements of worry and anxiety that are a part of typical development, there is also anxiety beyond the healthy developmental stages. When anxiety starts to interfere with life, learning, and experiences, it's time to intervene. The key to building a more resilient brain is impacting how the brain processes information and increasing the distance between your child and the cliff's edge of symptoms.

Pandemic Lessons

In over a decade at Brain Balance, I have witnessed the increasing rates of anxiety in kids. What initially felt like an infrequent question or concern from parents shifted over time to become a more common concern, with parents reaching out for help (beyond issues of attention and impulsivity). The data backs up my personal experience of the escalating trend, with the CDC reporting a three-point increase in the percentage of kids diagnosed with an anxiety disorder between 2003 and 2012, from 5.4% to 8.4% of kids ages six to seventeen.[1]

Then the pandemic hit, and the rates jumped again. In fact, the *Lancet* reported that since March 2020, anxiety in both kids and adults worldwide has increased an additional 26%, with women and young people particularly impacted.[2] It started with genuine fear of the unknown as this new pandemic spread worldwide and continued as the world adapted to massive changes in daily life. The sustained levels of heightened stress and the large changes, combined with an initial reduction in physical activity for kids as sports and activities shut down, created the perfect storm.

While we can't control the world around us, there are strategies we can use and development we can reinforce that can contribute to our kids' brains being more resilient in facing stress and anxiety and can perhaps provide a little more feeling of control in their lives.

Science Alert

The Oxford Languages dictionary defines *anxiety* as "a feeling of worry, nervousness, or unease, typically about an imminent event or something with an uncertain outcome."[3] **Anxiety is a feeling, but a feeling generated by activity in the brain.** The American Psychological Association adds physical elements to their definition of anxiety, describing it as "an emotion characterized by feelings of tension, worried thoughts and physical changes like increased blood pressure." They go on to state, "People with anxiety disorders usually have recurring intrusive thoughts or concerns. They may avoid certain situations out of worry. They may also have physical symptoms such as sweating, trembling, dizziness, or a rapid heartbeat."[4]

The important takeaway from these definitions is that anxiety is a feeling linked to physiological responses in the brain and body. To combat anxiety, we must do more than simply talk about the feelings. Strategies such as writing your worries down and placing them in a "worry jar" are good and beneficial—but they don't address the underlying mechanisms. To work toward preventing and minimizing anxiety, we need to strengthen how the brain processes information and the body's calming mechanisms in addition to the coping strategies that help manage those feelings.

To support a child struggling with anxiety, I find it helpful to understand what is happening in the brain and body when anxiety is triggered. This can help to guide strategies to minimize the effects.

It's important to note that what happens in the brain and body during anxiety overlaps very closely with what happens during anger. Both emotions result in a loss of control and involve increased stress hormones, increased activation of the emotional centers in the brain, and reduced activity in the higher-thinking parts of the brain. Psych Central, a mental health information and news website, differentiates anxiety from anger by explaining that anxiety comes from "fear and unease due to a perceived threat and anger is reactive" and occurs in a response to a threat paired with a feeling that you or someone else has been wronged.[5] **With anxiety, the brain and body responses are triggered due to your perception of a threat—real or imagined—or from thoughts about a possible threat.** "What if I fail this test?" "Will my friends include me at lunch today?"

Remember the vagus nerve we discussed in chapter 7? It is involved in anxiety too—it directs the activation or deactivation of calming mechanisms and impacts mood.[6] To understand the power of the vagus nerve, go back to the science section in chapter 7.

A loud noise startles your child and negative thoughts and worries start to kick in. Your child experiences a butterfly sensation in their tummy, sweating, an increased breathing and heart rate, tensing muscles, and a worsening mood. All this occurs without any conscious thought or awareness, shifting instantaneously due to the vagus nerve's response to a perceived threat. When this happens, the brain shifts into more of a survival mode. Your child can experience an *increase* in negative thoughts and emotions and a *decrease* in their ability to stop a thought or action, which can put that negative thought or worry on repeat in the brain.

An article published in the Harvard Medical School blog describes the body's stress response by explaining that two regions in the brain, the amygdala and the hypothalamus, work together to trigger a release of adrenaline. The adrenaline circulating in your system elevates your heart rate to push more blood to organs, muscles, and the brain to heighten your senses. There is also a release of glucose (blood sugar) to supply energy to all parts of the body. This chain of events is triggered so quickly that your visual system may not have even processed yet what is happening.[7]

Next, to sustain this heightened state of stress, the brain engages another chain of events to release cortisol. WebMD descibes cortisol as the body's main stress hormone that influences mood, motivation, and fear. Cortisol also increases blood sugar levels to provide more energy to the body.[8]

When the stressful event ends and the cortisol levels begin to drop, the calming mechanisms kick in through the vagus nerve, bringing you back calm, rested, and more focused.

This process takes a toll—it requires large amounts of fuel to support that initial and prolonged surge of stress and can leave you feeling depleted. Especially if that stress is sustained—like what we all experienced during the pandemic. With chronic stress the brain can be stuck in a state of constant high alert, a constant draining of fuel. The result: increased anxiety, a more negative and volatile mood, and a decrease in working memory and sustained attention.

Stress doesn't just deplete your resources; if persistent stress continues long enough there can be changes in both the function and structure of the prefrontal cortex and the amygdala. The prefrontal cortex is the region of the brain that contributes to our executive functions, working memory, self-regulation, and goal-directed behaviors. It is particularly sensitive to stress in infancy and adolescence.[9] Chronic stress can cause shrinking in the prefrontal cortex and an increase in activation of the amygdala, the region of the brain involved in experiencing emotions, making the brain even more sensitive to stress.[10] It's like a double whammy. The more stress and anxiety you face, the more stressed and anxious you feel, diminishing your resilience. This lowered threshold due to chronic stress is one of many factors that can contribute to anxiety as part of a trauma response. Someone who experienced trauma over a period of time can have a lower threshold, meaning their brain and body will tip over the edge into a state of anxiety more easily than others'.

That was a lot of science. The important takeaways are to understand *why* worry and anxiety make you feel and function in a certain way and the toll they take on you. Also, to understand the importance of minimizing chronic stress, lowering cortisol levels, and strengthening the vagal response to better regulate your state of relaxation. The good news? There are things you can do to help achieve these goals. Maturing aspects of the brain can help to reduce the frequency and intensity of feelings and reactions of anxiety.

Research shows that stimulating the vagus nerve can have an impact on mood and anxiety disorders,[11] and healthy lifestyle habits such as good sleep and exercise can help to reduce cortisol levels.[12] *Scientific American* states it simply, "When the vagus nerve is stimulated, calmness pervades the body: the heart rate slows and becomes regular; blood pressure decreases; muscles relax. When the vagus nerve informs the brain of these changes, it, too, relaxes, increasing feelings of peacefulness."[13] Combined, lowered cortisol levels, a stronger parasympathetic calming response, and more accurate sensory processing can make a big difference in a child's perception of and reaction to stress and anxiety.

Keep in mind that having fears and worries is a normal part of childhood development. This will present as developmental stages your child moves through. A general guideline is that normal anxiety is short-lived, does not interfere with your child's daily function or ability to perform tasks, and is something they move past with experience and understanding. If the anxiety is severe, frequent, and sustained for longer than several months, it's time to implement a plan of action, which can include strengthening the brain to minimize anxiety.

Infants and Toddlers

A baby's development will include times of reacting to or being fearful of many circumstances. Loud noises, heights, strangers, and separation from you are all considered normal fears for an infant or toddler. As your baby develops, their awareness and understanding of the world evolves, which will help to guide their future responses to these same events. In some instances, their expanding knowledge will *reduce* their fears, and in other instances it may *increase* their stress for a period of time.

Learning to understand what a new loud noise is can be an example of how learning and exposure help to reduce their stress and fear over time. The first time your child experiences fireworks, it's surprising—there are loud noises and bright colors raining down from the sky. With no previous experience of what fireworks are, that can be very frightening. Then, the next time they see fireworks, they know that while they are loud, they can also be fascinating to watch. They experienced this before and remained safe despite the noise, so there is no need to be afraid. (If they only see fireworks once a year, this can take a few times to understand and remember.)

Learning can also increase fear for a period of time. Separation anxiety is an example of this. When you leave the house and are gone for a while, your child will remember this experience. "When you go out the front door, I don't see you, and I don't like that." Experiencing that each time you leave you do come back will teach them that they will be okay, even when you leave. This is an example of moving through a stage of development.

The red flag for anxiety is when a child's learning or experience does not help them to move past their fear response. If every time they see fireworks, they become upset, this can indicate a disruption in their sensory system and how they process the noise, or a heightened fear response that is triggered too easily. If every time you leave they become inconsolable, and this continues for month after month without subsiding, this can be a sign that their nervous system is on high alert and their stress response is triggering too easily.

Anxiety Management Milestones for Infants and Toddlers

The lists below indicate events or things that may trigger developmentally appropriate anxiety at the following ages.

Seven to nine months:[14]
- Time away from caregivers
- Strangers; they begin to recognize faces at this age, and this creates the awareness of someone new

Up to two years:[15]
- Loud noises, heights, strangers

Three to four years:[16]
- Things that don't make sense, anything that isn't as it usually is— such as a grandparent who changed their hair color or a person in a costume
- Loud noises, such as thunder

- Imaginative things, such as ghosts, witches, monsters under the bed. This is due to a highly active imagination at this age.
- The dark or being alone at night, strange sounds, lights, or shadows on the wall
- Things they have seen on television or have read in books
- Scary dreams

Something to keep in mind (without guilt) is the importance of having time *away* from your child. And not just for self-care and survival for yourself, but to show your child that they are okay with a caregiver other than just you, and that you always come back.

As a new mom or dad, time away from your child can induce your own stress and anxiety; after all, you may have physically carried them for nine months and may be their primary source of nutrition initially. You are connected. I experienced this with Morgan, and because of my own stress I didn't leave often in the beginning, which made it harder for everyone involved down the road.

The first time I left the house without Morgan in tow was to run to the office supply store. I have no recollection of what I was doing, but I do remember how I felt. Anxious, rushed, phone in hand just in case. I hadn't been gone long when Doug called with a wailing Morgan in the background. Whatever it was I was trying to accomplish got set aside, and I raced back home feeling horrid—sweating, stressed, guilty, and even a little annoyed that I couldn't get something accomplished.

Hindsight is 20/20, and if I could go back and give advice to my younger self for this time period it would have been to get out—often. It will be stressful, hard, and uncomfortable in the beginning, but it will also be good. To show yourself, your partner, and your baby that you will all be okay with short times of separation.

For parents of infants during the pandemic, this scenario was heightened, as demonstrated by the photographer's one-year-old photo shoots you read about in the introduction. It was no longer just the stay-at-home parents who were rarely away from their child, but the work-from-home parents as well. Parents were left to either hire additional help, few of whom were willing to come into their home, or to juggle work and parenting on their own. Either way, it created very little opportunity to demonstrate to your infant that each time you leave, you will be back.

This was why the photographer stipulated that parents had to practice setting their child down on the floor and walking away—even just a few feet. They had to practice having someone new and different interact with their child, otherwise the photoshoot would be a bust.

Beyond conditioning through practice to facilitate learning, activating an infant's vagus nerve can provide a neurological approach to supporting feelings of calm and safety. The act of sucking and swallowing engages this bundle of nerves. Bottle-feeding a baby and holding them while their caregiver steps away or letting them suck on an infant chew toy if they are not hungry are ways to engage their calming mechanism.

The pandemic showed us that prolonged time at home with limited sensory exposure and experiences impacted kids' learning and development. They became familiar with the smells, sights, and sounds of home and immediate family, and not much else. While every day is a sensory experience for all humans, kids at home were utilizing the same pathways over and over, not building new ones through varied sensory exposures and experiences.

Another trigger for anxiety can be when a sensory experience is unknown or doesn't align with previous experiences, creating a reaction that may be beyond your child's ability to control.

An extreme example of this is the time Morgan jumped out and said "Boo!" to me. While this doesn't sound like a big deal—in that moment to me it was, and my knee-jerk reaction was big enough that she hasn't done it again.

I was coming into the house from a day at work, deep in thought and not paying attention to much of anything. Morgan heard the garage door open, so she knew I was pulling my car into the garage. She positioned herself behind the door and waited.

I opened the door and Morgan shouted, "Boo!" My nervous system kicked into instant fight or flight mode. I screamed and shouted, "Do not ever do that to me again!"

While my kids have certainly heard me shout many times before, it is normally an escalation over time, along the lines of, "you're not listening to me," "pick up your stuff," and the like. Not from happy to yelling in an instant. "Easy there, killer," was my husband's response, who had watched the whole thing. I completely over-reacted and my reaction was out of my control in that moment.

My expectation was a safe, calm, quiet environment. When I was met with surprise instead, my brain got scared. And reacted. Big. (Clearly I don't like it when people jump out to scare me.)

The same is true for kids experiencing something that is new, unexpected, or bigger than anticipated. A louder noise, firmer touch, stronger smell. All these can trigger the body's anxiety reaction. **We depend on the accuracy of our sensory perception to confirm our safety in our environment. Any disruption in this information will increase anxiety.** And remember, a disruption can be your brain and body experiencing the sensory event *differently* from others. Just because a noise or smell doesn't trigger stress in you doesn't mean it will be the same for your child. Just because you feel like you're not yelling doesn't mean your child will perceive it that way.

If any of this is sounding familiar, back up and review chapter 2. Sensory exposure and perception are necessary for learning and interpreting what is happening around you. Without strengthening sensory processing, calming anxiety will be an uphill battle—at all ages. And remember that the development of sensory pathways contributes to the development of the networks in the brain that support emotional regulation. Disruption in sensory processing is not just something that impacts kids who don't like tags on their clothing. It can be the teen who gets quiet at a school football game or large family gathering. It can be the parent who gets irritable when the kids are noisy in the car or feels drained after going to the mall. Or the toddler who prefers to remove their socks, shoes, or other pieces of clothing.

As your child experiences new things in life, be mindful of your tone and reactions. Before your child can regulate their own responses, they co-regulate through you. When something is new or different, they will take their cues from you on whether it is good or bad. Prior to an infant or toddler having a grasp of language and meaning, they can identify your tone of voice and when your reaction is different from the usual.

I am not saying that *you* are creating or dissipating your child's anxiety, but simply that as your child learns, you are helping to teach them whether something is safe or unsafe. Good or bad.

Fear of bees is a classic example of a child learning based on the tone and reaction from the adults around them. The first time a child sees a bee they have no reason to be afraid. It is tiny, makes a soft noise, and to a young child may be indistinguishable from a fly, which is harmless and seen more frequently (at least at our house) than bees.

But when a trusted caregiver shrieks, jumps up, and runs away, or points out frantically that a bee has landed on an arm, a very loud message is being sent. Bees are something to fear. Now the child may experience a fear of bees every time they see a bug flying or hear a buzzing noise.

Until your kids have their own frame of context for the things they experience in life, they will learn from yours. Even if bees trigger a stress response in you, by being mindful of your tone of voice, volume of reaction, and movements, you can help your child stay calm and relaxed.

Anxiety Management Activities for Infants and Toddlers

Review activities in chapter 2 as well.

Separation anxiety
- Begin by simply setting your child down but staying within their sight
- Build to moving out of their sight and returning, increasing the amount of time gradually
- Calm and soothe their nervous system through feeding them or giving them a teething toy to suck and chew on to engage the vagus nerve

Fear of strangers
- Expose your child to people outside your home; start at a distance with smiles and waves
- Ask the new people interacting with your child to keep their tone of voice calm and gentle

- Give your child time to observe the new person before expecting them to interact (don't just hand your baby to a grandparent they haven't seen in person in several months and expect this to go well; allow your child time to interact first within the safety of you holding them)

Fear of heights

- Do balance and proprioception activities (see chapter 1)

Elementary School Students

As kids get older, their fears will evolve with their awareness and imagination. Many kids at this age begin to understand that bad things can and do happen, so they may worry that someone they love may become sick or die. You are still their safety and comfort as they learn to explore the sometimes harsh realities of life.

Anxiety Management Milestones for Elementary Students

Five to six years:[17]

- Separation from you
  - May want to avoid school or sleepovers to stay with you to know you are safe
- Worry over getting lost or getting sick—as they become more aware that these things can happen, they worry
- Fear of monsters, witches, or other creatures or characters from movies or books
- Fear of the dark
- Nightmares and bad dreams
- Fire, wind, thunder, lightning—things that feel like they come out of nowhere; child is still learning cause and effect

Seven to eleven years:[18]

- Thinking becomes more concrete, but child still has a vivid imagination
- Fear of monsters, witches, or other creatures—that imagination is still hard at work!
- Fear of staying home alone—being away from you

- Worry about something happening to themselves and people or pets they love—starting to understand that death affects everyone, and is permanent
- Worry about rejection or not being liked by their peers
- Stress from everyday situations like school performance[19]

The elementary years can be a great time to teach and practice healthy breathing techniques. We all breathe all day, every day, but just because we do it doesn't mean we're doing it in the best possible way. In fact, most of us have pretty bad habits that lead to breathing that isn't as calming as it could be. Slouched posture and shallow breathing don't relax the body the way healthy breathing does.

Deep breathing—breathing into your belly—engages the diaphragm, a large muscle in your abdomen that sits below your lungs. When this muscle is engaged, especially when you exhale, it pushes the air from your lungs, activating the vagus nerve. Think of deep breathing as push-ups for the body's calming system. A study published in *Scientific Reports* demonstrated that just five minutes of deep, slow breathing can have an impact on the physiological stress that contributes to anxiety.[20]

Take a moment to notice your own breathing right now. Do you notice your chest or your stomach rising and falling? Far too many of us have the habit of shallow breathing, where the chest rises and falls. Especially if we're stressed out. When stressed, you may notice faster breathing and tense shoulders. When you're breathing shallowly, you work more of the smaller muscles that support breathing rather than the large diaphragm. Then, over time, this becomes habit. This contributes to stress and tension in your neck and shoulders, which then can exacerbate the shallow breathing.

Habits are hard to change, but it's possible. I recommend working together with your child on breathing and you'll both benefit.

You may be inclined to encourage your child to breathe deeply when they are crying or upset, but that isn't where I would start with improving breathwork. Instead, do this at a time when everyone is relaxed, calm, and happy. Working this into your bedtime routine is a great place to start. Have your child lie on their back with a hand placed on their chest and their other hand on their stomach. Have them breathe so that the hand on their stomach moves. This will give them both a physical and a visual cue to help them learn. Then have them take a couple of long, slow breaths.

The next step is teaching your kids why this simple activity is so powerful. You are teaching them how to exercise and engage their calming mechanisms. They can do this not only before bed to help them relax and drift off to sleep but anytime they want to feel more relaxed. Riding to school in the morning, sitting in class, hanging out with friends. There is never a bad time to breathe deeply to exercise relaxation. (And it doesn't have to be the loud inhale/exhale breathing to be effective—that would be awkward to do in class and with friends.)

Once this has become familiar and comfortable, encourage them to use this technique when they begin to feel irritated, stressed, or upset. Deep breaths can help stave off the body going into fight or flight and can help it recover from this state more quickly.

Ultimately, by working on breathing you are providing them a tool they can use to help themselves feel just a little bit better throughout life.

The goal is to do this so often it becomes automatic. Start by placing a few Post-it notes in strategic places. A note in the corner of your computer screen, on the dashboard in the car, the bathroom mirrors. Places you look often throughout the day. "BREATHE." This gentle reminder will cue you to remember to breathe deep into your belly and to take calming breaths throughout the day to stay calm and happy.

Breathing isn't the only way to activate the vagus nerve. This nerve bundle also controls many muscles in your face and throat. Laughing, humming, gargling, and even kissing are other ways to engage this nerve (the kissing recommendation is for you, not your kids!).

Gargling water when you brush your teeth, humming along to music in the car, or listening to a funny podcast are simple tricks to strengthen your level of calm and control.

Anxiety isn't logical, it's physiological, so reasoning with your child is not going to change or alter what is happening in the brain. Instead, acknowledge what is happening—"You're stressed, scared, uncomfortable, overwhelmed, unsure, or a combination of all those things. Right now your brain is telling you something. Your anxiety is a signal that your brain and body need a break to help reset back to calm. Are you listening, and what can we do based on what your brain is telling you?"

Years ago, we worked with a student at Brain Balance who had extreme anxiety around dust storms, to the point of having panic attacks. We live in North Carolina. Not a desert to be found that could produce a life-threatening dust storm. His mom had tried everything she could to educate her son about dust storms. Where they occur, the low prevalence, what to do if one occurs. Nothing helped. The boy could list all the statistics, he could look you in the eye one moment and tell you they don't happen here, and the next moment experience a panic attack, worried about the very thing he just told you wasn't possible.

This was an example of an incredibly bright boy, one who read for fun often and had a great imagination and gift for storytelling. He also had a very low threshold for stress and upsets, losing his temper or melting down more frequently than his fifth-grade peers. His assessment showed a persistent Moro reflex (the startle response), a brain that struggled to do tasks requiring separate functions at the same time, and heightened sensory perception. To sum it all up—his body was always on the verge of stress, so he needed to work harder to block out distractions to pay attention, and he struggled to do tasks that were more involved. His immature development resulted in a lack of control, which contributed to his anxiety; thoughts got stuck on repeat in his head and he couldn't get them to stop. Doing everyday tasks required a lot from him, depleting his fuel, pushing him closer to the edge of his personal cliff. When he got stressed or upset, his brain would go on a repeat cycle of doom and gloom, and the current subject was dust storms. (Remember the decreased prefrontal cortex and the increased amygdala activation? More negative mood and less control to stop the thoughts after persistent stress.)

Dust storms, or a lack of understanding about these storms, wasn't causing his anxiety. His immature, over-worked, overly sensitive system was causing the anxiety, and dust storms just happened to be the topic he thought about in that moment. His body was reacting to information as though he was quite young, yet his brain had the knowledge of an older student—a tough combination.

Throughout the program, as his brain matured, his moments of anxiety became fewer and far less intense. He also began to improve his ability to notice how he was feeling and talk about it. He shared that "when there was lots going on my brain would get the jitters." Lots of chaos and activity (sensory stimulation) elevated his stress, and then he had a hard time thinking clearly and regulating his mood and emotions. Things would go south quickly. This could happen with a busy day at school, times at home with siblings being noisy, or a parent yelling at him.

The trick to calming his anxiety was maturing how his brain took in and processed information, strengthening his calming systems, and activating his control. I also recommended he switch genres of reading for a while to something a little more lighthearted and fun than natural disasters.

A contributor to stress at this age is your child's increasing awareness of the world and the bad events that can take place. Cancer, car accidents, heart attacks, shark attacks, school shootings, the pandemic. Our world is full of scary realities, but as adults we (usually) have a greater capacity for understanding and processing this information and the prevalence of these events. (Although we all have our breaking point where the news and reality can be too much, too heavy, and, like our kids, we may need a moment to reset our mood and emotions.)

Know that your child's level of awareness and understanding is increasing, but they don't have the capacity of an adult to cope. They also still have the vivid imagination of youth, which can be a powerful combination. Worry, rumination, and a lack of perspective can elevate their fears quickly.

I vividly remember my own experience with this combination of awareness and fear as a child. When I was young, a local news story became a national headline when an eleven-year-old boy, Jacob Wetterling, was kidnapped from a small town in Minnesota. Not only was he similar in age to me, but he also lived in Minnesota. Jacob was with his brother and a friend biking home from renting a movie, something we also often did, when he was kidnapped.

Kidnapping was not something that had been real to me prior to this event. It was a term I knew, but the concept felt abstract, despite the warnings at school about stranger danger and avoiding white vans offering puppies or candy. Suddenly it was real, and every stranger and car was a potential kidnapper. I was scared to death to let my sisters out of my sight (which was the opposite of how I typically felt at this age). I remember becoming furious with my irresponsible mom one day while at the mall for her lackadaisical attitude (she isn't irresponsible in the least, it just felt that way in the moment). She was flipping through clothing on a rack, not paying attention to my sisters, who were chasing each other in and out of the racks of clothes; I was convinced that they would be snatched every moment I couldn't see them. They wouldn't listen, wouldn't hold my hand, and my mom was not helping at all.

Eventually my fear subsided as my frame of context expanded. Kidnapping *is* real, but it is also quite rare. There are also smart safety precautions you can take to minimize this from happening.

Know that it is normal for your kids to experience moments like this. Moments where the harsh reality of life becomes real. Acknowledge how they are feeling. Even if it's different from how you are feeling, it's what they are experiencing in the moment, which makes it real to them. Reassure them with facts and statistics and the things your family does to remain safe and healthy.

If their fear and anxiety escalate to the point of disruption, take a step back to consider what else could be contributing to a fight or flight response. Are they exhausted or over-stimulated? Do they have areas of possible immaturity in their development, making it harder for them to take in and process life's experiences, a lack of inhibitory control to stop their thoughts from playing on repeat? How do they tolerate sensory stimulation, and how strong are their executive functions that allow the brain to inhibit and move on from those negative thoughts?

Next, consider what you can do in the moment to activate their calming response and to provide them a sense of safety and calm. Gentle human touch through a hug or a snuggle on the couch. Deep breathing to enhance a feeling of calm and engage the vagal system. Movement and exercise to help shift gears in the brain and move past the worry or upset.

You may be asking, if a child has experienced trauma, how does that impact their experience with stress and anxiety, and do these same tactics apply?

Remember that cliff's edge we talked about in chapter 7? Think of trauma as bringing the brain one giant step closer to the cliff's edge. People who have experienced trauma can have a brain that is locked at or near the edge of fight or flight. Which means little to nothing can tip them over the edge, producing symptoms of anxiety.

With the kids I've worked with over the years, I've seen over and over how trauma freezes aspects of development, creating immaturities. I knew this in theory, but that theory became real to me as I sat across from a single mom discussing her child's evaluation. I pointed out that even though her child was ten years old, in function after function she was presenting in line with what would be expected of a six-year-old's development. With tears in her eyes, the mom shared the trauma that had occurred at that age. While her daughter's body continued to develop, several of her developmental functions remained behind. Her ability to pay attention, process information, and do more complex, involved tasks remained stuck. Counseling was needed and had been in place for years. Maturing her brain would not be a replacement for therapy but an enhancement. We often see that as aspects of development mature, kids (and adults) can become more able to apply the practices and strategies learned in therapy to their lives (as Doug said, first neurology, then psychology).

Through exercising this young lady's infant reflexes and building core strength, coordination, sensory perception, and timing began to mature beyond the six-year-old level—in both her emotional maturity and ability to pay attention and regulate her behaviors. The trauma will always be a part of her past, and she continued to work with a professional to support her healing, but strengthening her brain provided her with increased maturity and a decrease in her persistent anxiety.

So the answer is *yes*, when working with someone who has a history of trauma, you can use the same tactics to contribute to a process of creating and supporting a more resilient brain. I also recommend you work directly with a therapist who specializes in supporting these concerns.*

Anxiety Management Activities for
Elementary School Students

Refer back to activities in chapter 7 as well.

Strategies for breathwork

- Breathe with hand on chest and belly to learn to breathe deep into the stomach
- Practice slow, intentional breathing—there are a variety of recommendations for timing for inhale/exhale. A deep breath in for a five count, then a five count or longer exhale has been shown to be calming.
- Place Post-it notes in visible places for frequent reminders to breathe this way throughout the day. This can help create healthy habits of deep belly breathing.
- Practice implementing breathing at times of calm and relaxation. Then begin to use this strategy when starting to feel stressed or agitated. Finally, begin using this strategy once an upset has occurred to help move past the fight or flight response more efficiently.
- Be aware of posture; put shoulders back to help open up the chest to support healthy breathing.
- Stretch to open up the chest; it can feel great and help to support good posture
  - Lie on a yoga ball on your back with arms extended out
  - Raise an arm like you're going to wave, place the forearm on the wall, and gently lean into the stretch; this can also help to open the chest

---

*Reminder: This book is intended as an informative guide for those wishing to learn more about supporting their child's development and well-being. It is not intended to replace, countermand, or conflict with advice given to you by your own physician. The ultimate decisions concerning your care should be made between you and your doctor.

- Do front plank exercises, push-ups, or other exercises to engage the upper back muscles; this can help to support posture by pulling shoulders back to open up the chest

Additional ways to engage the vagus nerve

- Gargling (water is fine)
- Humming
- Laughter
- Kissing (when age- and situation-appropriate)
- Facial massage

Ways to support a child's expanding awareness of the world

- Acknowledge that what your child is feeling is real to them; do not discredit it or blow off their feelings or emotions
- Have frank and honest conversations with your kids, be real and honest but not alarming
- Discuss the things you do to remain safe and well

Consider the state of your child's brain and
body during times of anxiety

- Are they tired, hungry, or in an overwhelming sensory environment?
- Have they been asked to do something they don't feel equipped to do? Is there a way you can help them feel supported or equipped in the moment?

Middle School and High School Students

If your child is middle school or high school age, don't start this chapter here; back up and read the section for elementary ages as well as the tips and explanations that apply to older kids and adults.

There is so much happening for teens that can increase stress, making them more susceptible to anxiety. Teens are experiencing peer pressure; juggling school, sports, and friendships; and deciding what to do and where to go after high school on top of distractions and hormones. Additionally, they often have social media and the constant reminders and pressure that accompany this aspect of life. And those are just a few of the logical stressors that can contribute to their anxiety. Remember, anxiety is based on how their brains and bodies perceive things, which may not be logical to you.

They can also be experiencing anxiety based on how they feel they compare to others—from physical appearance to grades, fitting in with friends, and romantic relationships. These are all additional stressors that can trigger anxiety at any age but can be heightened at this time of life.

Anxiety Management Milestones for Middle School and High School Students

Twelve and older:[21]

As your teen continues their path toward independence, their dependence on you starts to lessen and their peer group takes on larger importance in their life. At this age these are things that can cause worries and stress:

- What their peers are thinking of them
- Performance in school—worry about grades, exams, and next steps in life
- Events they see on the news—school shootings, getting sick, themselves or someone they care about dying
- Talking to parents about important personal issues—while they strive toward independence, they still want to make you proud and care about what you think, even if it doesn't always feel that way
- Fear of missing out—of being excluded or left out of events and activities with friends

Catastrophizing. What a great word to describe a horrible feeling. We've all been there—that moment where your brain jumps to the worst-case scenario and blows things out of proportion. Catastrophizing happens when the brain is under high levels of stress. Thoughts will often revert to the past—"that one time I was late and forgot my pencil and my teacher yelled at me, and now she hates me, and I'm going to be late again, this is the worst day ever, and I'll never pass this class."

A whirlwind of bad thoughts and feelings. In fact, thoughts jumping to the past and going negative, *really* negative, can be a red flag that the brain is in a state of catastrophizing. The result is a brain that has a harder time focusing, controlling behaviors, and regulating mood and emotions, and that struggles to look ahead to plan and address the moment.

While this can happen at any age, your teen may experience catastrophizing during this time as the pressure of school mounts—they may be trying to decide what they want to do after high school and feeling like they need to decide now what they want to do for the rest of their lives. Juggling increasingly busy schedules that may include sports, activities, homework, and jobs on top of finding time for friends can feel like a lot. This age also has a large focus on figuring out who they are and how they fit into the groups and peers around them. Being excluded can feel devastating, and social media provides a level of awareness we didn't experience at their age.

Like trying to use logic and reasoning with a toddler in the throes of a meltdown, mid-catastrophizing is *not* the time to use logic with your teen. This is another version of an upset, and reasoning just isn't going to happen. Instead, help your child recognize when this is happening and what it signals. The brain is on overload and is experiencing high stress. To break this moment, the brain needs support and time to reset. Save the longer conversation and logic for later when they are calm and more focused.

In the beginning you'll need to guide your resistant and negative child through navigating their way out of this moment. They may be taller than you at this age, but as a primary caregiver you are still helping them to co-regulate until they can do it on their own.

Teach your child to go through a mental inventory—like a preflight checklist. "If I'm feeling this way my brain needs something—what can I do to help?" "I don't feel like I have the resources to handle this moment—what is it that would help? A friend or parent to talk to? Taking a break to relax? Have I gotten enough sleep, eaten enough? What can I do right now to feel better? What can I do over the next twenty-four hours to feel better?" (Refer to the activities section in this chapter for a list of ideas.)

Drew will have catastrophizing moments when he is exhausted and overwhelmed. With a priority on spending as much time as possible outside with buddies shooting hockey pucks or fishing, he will put homework and studying out of his mind. Which means Sunday night when it's getting late, and he remembers his list of assignments he hasn't done, his mood can take a quick turn. If he's stressed for an upcoming history test he hasn't studied for and can't find his notes for, if he is frustrated with his math homework, has a science lab sheet due, and is drained from hours of physical exercise and late nights, that is not the time for productive studying or even a conversation. "I hate this class, when in life am I *ever* going to need to know about this, he's such a bad teacher, I already got a bad quiz grade, so I know I'm going to fail [despite his history of being an honor roll student—but remember no logic right now], blah, blah, blah."

Ten p.m. is not the time to break out a list of subjects to work on for Monday morning. It's also not the time for more exercise. Telling him to take deep breaths in this moment will only earn me a look. In this moment, having Drew write down what he needs to do and having him pick the *one* thing that is most urgent is a start (his response is that it is all urgent, and he'll fail everything if he doesn't get it all done *right then*). If his history class is first the next day I would have him do his work for that one class. Then go to bed with an alarm set earlier than normal for the next day (and a reminder to breathe deeply to help fall asleep). The next morning is a better time to tackle the math homework, and then he can see that he will have time over lunch and study hall to finish the last assignment. Minor crisis managed. Sort of.

And after an unpleasant end to a Sunday, you can believe Doug and I will make sure there are fewer late nights and more time spent on homework earlier in the weekend next time.

While Drew's homework procrastination is a small example of catastrophizing, kids today are experiencing very real and difficult scenarios that in the moment can feel monumental. Instilling the awareness of this experience and practicing strategies to move past this moment with small incidents and upsets can help set the stage for healthy strategies when the upsets and tough moments get tougher. Teach kids that their brain is making things seem even worse, and with some time, a plan, or even someone to help you with a plan—a parent, friend, or therapist—they *will* feel better.

Beyond understanding catastrophizing, it's also critical to remember the lack of impulse control in anyone when exhausted or stressed, and in those with conditions such as ADHD. Reduced inhibitory control from immature development can lead to little problems, such as trouble paying attention, and also major trouble, such as rushing to make big decisions.

My dad, a retired colonel, has a fellow veteran friend who counsels military suicide survivors. He shared with my dad that every single person who attempted suicide by jumping off a bridge said that as they were falling, they regretted it. Think about that for a moment. A potentially impulsive decision being made at a time when the brain is stuck on a loop of negativity and hopelessness.

Let your kids know that what they are feeling right now is hard, but it will pass. As bad as it feels right now, tomorrow, a week from now, and a month from now it won't feel as bad as it does in this moment. The hope is that by teaching this with smaller incidences at a young age, kids are better equipped to face the bigger, heavier moments that will inevitably happen throughout life. The online or in-person bullying. The picture you regret taking that gets shared around the school. The girlfriend who breaks up with you, leaving you feeling alone. The pandemic showed us all that life will throw you unimaginable curveballs. Sometimes your brain tells you a story even worse than reality, but with a plan to identify and disrupt the catastrophizing and strengthen the brain's inhibitory control, you can push through to the other side of the upset.

The teenage years are a great time to both continue to strengthen the brain and drive home the power of exercise. It is so much more than cardiovascular health—exercise also impacts your mood, attention, energy, memory, and impulse control. Learning how and when to implement exercise at a young age will create a healthy, lifelong habit.

Physical activity can be used to engage and exercise the calming effect of the vagus nerve. Each time you exercise to the point of going breathless and elevate the heart rate, the vagus nerve kicks in. Doing interval training is a way to engage this system repeatedly. There are so many ways to quickly spike heart rate—burpees, jump rope, stair sprints, or just sprinting. No fancy gear or equipment needed. Get your body moving and you'll exercise not only your muscles but your parasympathetic nervous system as well.

Exercise is a double positive for feeling good. Not only does exercise *reduce* your levels of cortisol, the stress hormone, but it can also trigger a release of endorphins that contributes to feelings of happiness.[22] While there are many theories on how much exercise is needed for various goals, endorphins have been shown to increase after thirty minutes of moderate exercise.[23] And doing exercise in a group setting rather than alone was shown to release *more* endorphins in a small study on synchronized activity.[24]

When I find myself in a negative headspace, I know the best thing I can do to turn things around is go for a run—for the reasons mentioned and more. Providing myself some free-range thinking time where thoughts bounce from topic to topic can help process thoughts and feelings and provide beneficial brainstorming. (Remember the default network from chapter 4.) When feeling stressed or anxious, we often engage in activities to avoid our own thoughts, as they can be uncomfortable. As adults we grab our phones and aimlessly scroll, turn on the TV to immerse ourselves in another world, stay buried in work, or reach for a cocktail. We can help support our kids in creating healthy lifestyle habits that provide them comfort and practice with free-thinking time. Time when they are not actively engaged in a task that occupies their thoughts, so they learn to be alone with their own minds.

If I don't have time to go for a run, I'll take just a minute to do some squat jumps. Engaging large muscle groups, core muscles, and elevating your heart rate helps to clear your mind and re-energize or refocus your thoughts. Keep in mind that when your kids are feeling down, anxious, or upset, it can be one of the hardest times to motivate them to exercise. Encourage them to start small—do lunges down the hallway as they head to the bathroom. Do a few push-ups or sit-ups between episodes of the show they're binge-watching.

When it comes to teaching these strategies to your kids, you'll feel like a broken record, but one of these days it may sink in. And then just try to bite your tongue instead of shouting "I told you so" when they notice how good they feel after moving.

Rather than nagging your kids to exercise when they're anxious, model this yourself or point out the difference exercise makes for a sibling or friend.

"I'm so stressed today, I'm going to start the day with a run so I can focus later." "Notice what a great mood your brother is in after hockey. Exercise makes the brain feel so good!" "I'm feeling stuck with my writing, so I'm taking a break to move and turn my brain back on."

Our pandemic response involved cutting teens off from their in-person social interactions and isolating them at home. This went against the nature of their developmental needs and contributed to escalating rates of anxiety and depression. I'm not sharing this to cause guilt—rather to build awareness and intentionality about the importance of peer connection in middle and high school.

A friend in California witnessed the impact of the pandemic on her daughter Ella. A ninth grader when the pandemic hit, Ella shifted from being a high school soccer player with a bursting social life to a recluse in her room. Since her only way to connect with friends was through Snapchat, FaceTime, and other social media apps, her parents let this happen without time limits. She saw when friends were getting together, even though her family wasn't getting together with others at this time. Her mood spiraled, and her anxiety escalated.

My friend shared that with both parents working from home, they were all home, all the time, but not really connecting. The younger kids seemed to be doing fine, going outside to ride bikes and play, so they were still getting activity outside the house.

After an explosive conversation after dinner one night, my friend realized something needed to change—they needed to get Ella moving and active again. The family started to take time in the evening and on weekends to get out of the house and enjoy nature. Mountain biking, kayaking, hiking. Anything they could think of. While everyone in the family enjoyed the activities (most of the time), Ella was still struggling. They had her start to work with an online therapist, which helped them realize how desperately Ella needed in-person time with friends.

They connected with a family they knew who lived nearby who was also continuing to isolate at home. They decided to work together on finding opportunities for the girls to get together in ways they all felt comfortable doing.

"That first day Ella came home from spending a few hours outside with her friend, I cried. I hadn't realized how long it had been since I had seen a genuine smile on her face." My friend shared this story on a friends' group video call. After she talked about Ella's struggle, the other moms shared various iterations of the same theme. Cutting off social interactions was hurting us all, especially our teenagers. To quote another friend, "Family time is great, but this much family time with no friend time is just not natural at this age!"

The combination of less sensory exposure and less physical activity paired with prolonged stress brought out underlying anxiety in people of all ages around the world (remember that prolonged stress lowers your threshold for what can trigger anxiety). To counter this effect we need to find ways to bring positive emotions back into the brain and activate the prefrontal cortex for inhibitory control to more effectively stop negative thoughts and actions.

Social interactions and dynamics are so important at this age—with or without a pandemic. It is on us to help kids learn about themselves and build relationships outside their families. Laughter, fun, and belonging are all great feelings that contribute to our sense of well-being and happiness, but there is also a calming benefit to the brain and body with positive connections and face-to-face social interactions. A 2013 study out of the University of North Carolina discussed a feedback loop that demonstrated an increase in vagal activation through experiencing positive emotions as a result of positive social connections.[25]

Anxiety Management Activities for Middle School and High School Students

Review activities sections for younger ages as well as the activities in chapters 2, 7, and 9.

Things you can do in the moment to break the cycle of anxiety (depending on the timing and environment)
- Deep breathing, meditation, or yoga
- Eat (it will take roughly twenty minutes for the fuel to kick in and support improved focus)

- Engage the brain in a different task that occupies thoughts
- Spend time with a good friend
- Make a to-do list and highlight only what needs to be done right then
- Exercise
  - ○ Interval training for exercising the brain's calming response
  - ○ Group exercise to enhance endorphin release and spend positive time with friends
  - ○ Moderate exercise for at least thirty minutes to release endorphins to help elevate mood
- Journal
- Sleep (see chapter 9 to learn more about good sleep hygiene and needs by age)
- Use minimal caffeine—caffeine increases cortisol, the stress hormone in the body
- Stay aware of sugar consumption and how you feel—remember that blood sugar levels and cortisol, the stress hormone, are related. Sugar intake can drive up the release of stress hormones.
- Take probiotics—gut bacteria has been shown to influence the vagus nerve, as elements of the nerve involve communication from the gastrointestinal tract to the brain.[26]

Signs That Indicate Improvement

As a parent it is often easier to notice the onset of something than the slow dissipation of symptoms. Improvements with anxiety will be slow and gradual over time. You'll begin to notice your child moving through the moment faster and having fewer times of anxiety. You'll know you're really on the right track when your child is able to begin to verbalize how they are feeling and the strategies they are using to positively impact their feelings and ability to do what is needed. Fewer complaints of stomachaches and headaches and fewer excuses to try to get out of attending events and activities can also be a positive sign that your child is beginning to experience a reduction in their anxiety.

9

. . . .

OPTIMIZE WELL-BEING

I don't know a single parent (and I know a lot of parents) who hasn't worried about their child's well-being at some point, especially after these past few years. The isolation, changes, and stress have layered on top of the natural growing pains of development. Growing up comes with a variety of emotions and experiences, and adding the pandemic into the mix has made these past few years harder in so many ways, yet taught us so many valuable lessons. The number of kids struggling was already escalating, and then the pandemic hit, furthering the negative impact. The Seattle school district saw such a worsening of mental health and behavioral disorders among its students that it had to increase staffing to support them. The school district believes that the sharp increase of social media consumption contributed to these worsening behaviors and mental health concerns. As a result, the district filed a lawsuit against the tech companies behind the mega social media platforms of Instagram, TikTok, YouTube, Facebook, and Snapchat.[1]

As parents, when we're worried we lose sleep; we talk with spouses, friends, and other parents; and we scour the internet. We want to know if what we are observing in our kids is typical; we want to know what it means and how to help our kids.

Pandemic parents are not the only parents to watch their kids and wonder and worry. Life and development are complex, and every brain has opportunities for improvement, at every age. Parenting is hard, and the honest answer is that some kids are more difficult to parent than others. This doesn't make them bad kids, nor their parents bad parents. But when a child struggles with impulse control, managing their emotions, staying on task, or reading social cues, it can make a hard situation even more difficult. And while all those scenarios will increase levels of stress at home, nothing will weigh on your parent heart like concern for your child's well-being.

Note to Parents

It isn't realistic to expect that all moments will be happy ones. Stress and challenges naturally arise throughout all lives, our kids' included. The human experience is a dynamic one and has a full spectrum of moods and emotions. Equipping our kids to face life's ups and downs and challenges is the goal. To support achieving that goal, helping kids learn to identify how they're feeling and functioning and teaching them healthy ways to handle life's stressors can facilitate overall well-being.

My goal is to show you how to help your kids to recognize how they're feeling and what they can do to support the brain to help put their mindset and well-being in the best possible position. This isn't about being happy; it's about being *resilient*. Resilience is defined by the Oxford dictionary as "the capacity to recover quickly from difficulties; toughness." And we all need as much of that as possible.

Pandemic Lessons

As you've learned throughout this book, each brain has a threshold for how much it can tolerate, and when that threshold has been exceeded, there are always consequences. When the brain is stressed and/or challenged for prolonged periods, has short periods with high stress, or reaches sensory overload, it impacts all the executive and cognitive functions: attention, memory, cognitive flexibility, and inhibition. It also impacts mood and emotions, resulting in outward displays of fatigue, irritability, and anxiety; losing control of emotions and behaviors is not uncommon. You or your child may feel more negative, more anxious, more stressed, and less effective in what you're trying to accomplish. In this state, you're more likely to make poor choices that result in even further negative feelings of shame, regret, and guilt.

These years of sustained stress and change have stretched the limits of what we can handle and have resulted in massive increases in diagnosed—and undiagnosed—mental wellness concerns. This time has taught us more about what stresses and challenges the brain. On a positive note, this period has also demonstrated that the brain can change and what it takes to help move mental health in a better direction. Applying what you learn in this book can help you get your child's well-being back on track.

Science Alert

We classify our mood and emotions as feelings. Science has shown that those feelings are neurons that fire in a particular pattern. Feelings are a network of connections that link multiple regions of the brain and provide sensations, context, and content to what is happening around us.[2] Our feelings originate in the brain. Feeling calm and relaxed on a sunny day at the beach is a pattern of connections, just like a physical action such as a jumping jack is a pattern of connections.

For decades, the focus of mental health and well-being researchers and doctors has been on understanding the body's chemistry. When someone is experiencing a mental health crisis or concern, the doctors often reference the term *chemical imbalances*, then address the chemistry through medication. This approach is often paired with therapy to help identify and process thoughts and emotions and to provide helpful coping strategies. While this approach has been helpful for many, further evolution of the approach, and additional options, are needed. Recent science is beginning to move beyond the mental health theory of chemical imbalance as researchers make advances to better understand the mechanisms in the brain that contribute to our well-being (and hopefully provide advancements and interventions). In fact, recent research published in the journal *Molecular Psychiatry* directly questions the "serotonin hypothesis" of depression, which is part of the chemical imbalance theory. This long-standing theory holds that when a person is experiencing depression, or dysregulation in mood, it is due to not enough serotonin being present in the system (serotonin is a neurotransmitter that activates certain neurons and pathways). The recent research claims there isn't a strong enough link between serotonin levels and depression to support this long-held theory.[3] Dr. Thomas Insel, the former director for the National Institute for Mental Health, has been a vocal advocate for challenging the mental health field to try to better understand the impact of genetics and brain connectivity to guide improvements in interventions and support.[4]

Similarly, positive self-talk has long been seen as one way to impact the patterns of your thoughts. "Think positive to feel positive" can be easier said than done. It is true that positive thoughts elicit positive emotions by triggering those pathways. But understanding more about the brain allows us to make it easier to access and strengthen the pathways that produce positive thoughts. Positive self-talk is harder to do when your brain doesn't have what it needs to perform at its best. We need to understand what the brain needs in order to be more able to access the pathways in the brain that support positive mood, emotions, and thoughts. We need the neurological ability to apply the psychological approach. In this chapter we'll discuss how to ensure the brain has what it needs to both access and improve the pathways that support our mood, emotions, and thoughts.

If you're feeling tired, hungry, or stressed, all the positive self-talk in the world won't change the fact that your brain is running low on resources, feeling more negative, and having a harder time accessing higher-level functions. In fact, when you're at this point, it's incredibly difficult to engage in positive self-talk and actually mean it. **If you start by being rested, well-fed, emotionally fulfilled, and motivated, your brain will naturally and easily access and utilize those positive self-talk emotional pathways. So you must first make sure your brain has what it needs. This will make it possible to have more positive thoughts that will in turn encourage feelings of happiness and fulfillment.**

The goal of this chapter is to show you how to do just that—how to give your child's brain what it needs so it can achieve a rested, energized, and motivated state. There are daily strategies you can implement to increase your child's threshold before they reach the point of no return, to keep them happier for longer and help them bounce back faster when they tip over the cliff's edge.

The strategies we'll discuss are universal to all ages and stages of development, but they require different approaches to implement at different ages.

Be sure to read all three sections of this chapter to learn the tips and tricks for a more resilient brain.

Infants and Toddlers

Clearly, positive self-talk isn't the focus of supporting infants (but can benefit the new and exhausted parents). At this age a great place to focus is on creating healthy routines and patterns to support development. These include sleep, face-to-face interaction, sensory play, movement, healthy eating, and more sleep. I do realize that this can be easier said than done and that accomplishing this list can vary greatly from child to child, even in the same home. Think of these guidelines as overarching goals you are striving toward, not as a checklist that needs to be perfect each day.

Well-Being Milestones for Infants and Toddlers

Sleep recommendations by age:[5]
- Four to twelve months: 12–16 hours
- One to two years: 11–14 hours
- Three to five years: 10–13 hours

Protein recommendations by age:[6]
Consult your pediatrician for recommendations specific to your child. This information is meant as a general reference guide only.
- Zero to four months: 8 grams per day
- Four to twelve months: 12 grams per day
- One to four years: 14 grams per day
- Four to five years: 19 grams per day

Screen time recommendations by age:[7]
- Zero to eighteen months: *No* screen time except for video chatting
- Eighteen months to five years: Less than an hour a day of quality educational content with a parent or caregiver

I love the phrase "Getting back to basics is the simplest way to find calm in the chaos." Sleep. Eat. Exercise. These are the cornerstones for a resilient brain—for everyone.

There's nothing better than a good night's sleep where you wake up refreshed and energized. Did you know that the average person spends 229,961 hours of their life sleeping? That equates to roughly twenty-six years, or one-third of your life.[8] Sleep is a big deal. In addition to all the time spent asleep, we spend an additional seven years *trying* to sleep—tossing, turning, and drifting in and out of sleep.[9]

What is it about sleep that's so crucial for our brain and body? While you sleep, there's a lot going on in your brain and body in terms of maintenance, organization, and energy.

In the *maintenance* element of sleep, the brain gets rid of debris and toxic waste. In fact, *Scientific American* describes sleep as the "deep clean."[10] It's believed that oscillations in blood flow linked to non-REM sleep spread cerebrospinal fluid throughout the brain to help flush out neural waste. During this phase of sleep, cellular repair also takes place. Researchers are realizing just how critical this cleaning and repair time is to healthy brain function. A big focus of ongoing research is understanding how prolonged disruptions in sleep contribute to cognitive decline and disease. Apply this concept to your kids—a sleep deficit impacts cognition. Staying up late to study can backfire on the ability to learn and retain information for our older kids, and disrupted or reduced sleep could potentially impact the cognitive development of our little ones.

The *organizational* element of sleep also appears to be connected to the non-REM oscillations that trigger electrical activity. During sleep, the brain reviews information and activity taken in throughout the day and decides what to keep and what to clear out. This process is called *consolidation*. It's how recent experiences get transformed into long-term memories.[11] Essentially, the brain doesn't store everything. The more intense the experience, or the more connections that were made in learning, the more likely the brain will consolidate this information so you can access it days, months, and years later. That's why learning is more powerful when you engage the senses and movement; more connections make information more likely to be stored in memory. This means lack of sleep can disrupt the efficacy of memory.

Sleep rejuvenates our energy through a release of molecules and hormones that prepare us for the next day. Sleep supports the executive and cognitive functions of memory, attention, cognitive flexibility, and inhibition. Sleep also supports our emotional regulation and mental health. While executive functions and cognitive functions look different in an infant and a toddler, they're still there, as seen in their ability to focus on a toy, listen while you speak, and cooperate. **While you sleep, brain activity increases in the areas that regulate emotions.**[12] **When you're well rested, your brain can respond in a more adaptive manner. When you're tired, you're far more likely to overreact—at any age.**

To sum it up, sleep is required for the brain to function, and it's important at all ages and stages of life. It becomes even more important during times of development and learning. The hard work and learning that happen during the day are less effective if you don't get quality sleep to organize and store those new connections.

Our little ones make it easy for us to know when it's time for them to sleep. There's a steep decline in their mood and behavior. In their own way, they're communicating their needs to you—sometimes very loudly and dramatically. No doubt you've already observed this through a shutdown in their ability to focus, think, make good decisions, communicate, and control their emotions and reactions.

Creating healthy sleep habits is key, and sticking to those habits and routines sets the whole family up for success. It's so easy for parents to get caught up in times of fun on vacation or at a celebration or party and to deviate from the routine. But there's always a price to pay.

To me, vacations, holidays, and times of fun are when it is even *more* important to stick to a sleep routine. These are times of sensory overload, and if you want your child to be able to enjoy the experience with less chance of a meltdown, sleep is simply critical.

The next basic element to consider is fuel for the brain and body. Fuel comes from what we eat, and I know that feeding toddlers and kids can be hard. Parents can feel a lot of emotions in the process of feeding their children—feelings of guilt if your child is a picky eater, images of quality family time that are shattered by power struggles that play out over a plate of meat and vegetables. These add stress to fueling our kids adequately, let alone well.

I want to remind you about the importance of offering your kids varied nutrients, but don't feel bad if your child isn't there yet. Picky eating is real, and I do not subscribe to the theory that "if they get hungry enough, they will eat it." That isn't always true. Not everyone feels hunger the same way. Feeling hunger is an interoceptive ability to sense and feel your own body and know what its signals mean. Picky eating is also a natural part of development. Check the activities section of this chapter for a few tips and tricks to help with picky eating. Also check out the Instagram account @kids.eat. in.color, which is dedicated to realistic and healthful strategies to support feeding your kids.

Next, let's dig into one of the reasons why lots of different nutrients are needed to support a growing brain and body. The foods we eat provide the fuel that is converted into energy. But it's easy to forget that what we eat provides the necessary tools for growth. Amino acids are required for building proteins, hormones, and muscle, as well as regulating immune function, digestion, neurotransmitters, and so much more.[13] The body produces many, but not all, of the amino acids we need, which means we need to get the rest from the foods we eat. If we're not consuming foods that contain these amino acids, the body will be missing key building blocks that support critical functions and development.

Animal proteins like meat, eggs, and poultry contain the amino acids we don't produce in our bodies.[14] You can also obtain these amino acids from eating a variety of beans, nuts, seeds, whole grains, and vegetables.

It's not always easy to convince your kids to eat protein, beans, seeds, and vegetables. Between the color, texture, and taste, our kids often want to avoid these foods. Instead, they all too often gravitate to dairy, carbs, fried foods, and sweets. In fact, chicken nuggets, macaroni and cheese, cheese pizza, and goldfish crackers make up the bulk of a lot of kids' diets. If your child isn't ready to eat healthy foods, don't give up. Continue to include healthy foods on their plate at each meal, but then back them up with nutritional supplements to ensure they have the nutrients they need. I'm a "food first" person, meaning my goal is to provide my kids and myself all the nutrients needed through foods rather than supplements. Good-quality food is the ideal way to receive nutrients, but if that isn't happening for now, defer to high-quality supplements (you get what you pay for when it comes to supplements, so I recommend not going cheap here).

When it comes to fuel, not all sources are created equal. Picture the moment: you're out with the family for the day, and your little one starts to become whiny and cranky. You can feel the meltdown approaching. There's no opportunity for a nap, so your next go-to is food. You dig in your giant mom- or dad-purse to grab whatever you can find.

You ask, "Do you want a peanut butter sandwich [that's now mashed from being buried in your purse] or a cookie?"

While both options will distract your child while they eat and provide a boost to their energy, one will help sustain their mood for longer, and the other will have you revisiting this same scenario much faster. Can you guess which is which?

Carbohydrates are the primary source of energy for the brain and body.[15] Sugar also provides a quick energy source that can boost mood and energy, but it's a fast-burning fuel that results in an energy crash once that fuel has been depleted. Protein and healthy fats—such as those found in nuts, avocado, and coconut oil—are slow-burning fuels that can be combined with carbs to provide a more even-keeled energy for longer. Kids need a combination of all three elements—carbohydrates, fats, and protein—for energy and to support their brain as well as their growth, mood, and behavior.[16]

As young parents, my husband and I quickly learned that our daughter Morgan needed a consistent protein intake. A generally sweet and easy-going child, she'd become whiny when her fuel levels dipped. Through trial and error, we realized that twenty minutes after consuming protein she would be back to her sweet self. The second she started to become teary or whiny, my husband and I would look at each other and ask, "What and when did she eat last?" Simply eating anything through the day wasn't enough; we needed to ensure she was consuming protein and carbs to best support her mood and energy. We had to get creative to sneak protein in throughout the day, but it benefited the whole family when we did. It was easier to incorporate protein at mealtimes than in snacks, but it was worth the effort to impact her mood. Protein smoothies, protein powder sprinkled in her oatmeal, nut crackers with hummus, nut butter on anything—bananas, bread, rice cakes.

We got creative and brought protein snacks everywhere we went. It was our survival tactic to keep Morgan happy and cooperative and us sane.

In addition to the importance of nutrients and consistent energy sources, a chapter on well-being would not be complete without acknowledging the importance of gut health and the gut–brain connection. This has been a large focus of research in the last decade, with studies indicating a correlation between gut health, mood, and mental well-being.[17] According to research from Johns Hopkins Medicine, changes in the gut's enteric nervous system, the elements of your nervous system that are located in the walls of your gut lining, may send signals to the brain that impact mood changes.[18] A review of many studies that looked at the gut–brain connection and mood, published in *Frontiers in Psychiatry*, found that gut microbiota can influence mood and that mood can influence gut microbiota. Additionally, the study found pre- and probiotics can impact mood.[19] This is an area of study that is rapidly growing, increasing our understanding of the impact of gut health and expanding our options for help.

The third basic strategy to support brain well-being is exercise, which for little ones is simply play. Most people are well versed in the importance of exercise for overall health, so let's talk a bit more about the impact exercise has on the brain and on mood.

Exercise helps to stimulate production of brain-derived neurotrophic factor (BDNF), a substance produced in the body that's needed to form new connections in the brain and ultimately contributes to learning and cognitive performance.[20] BDNF also contributes to the protection of the brain. The brain has a unique layer of protection called the blood-brain barrier. This layer keeps the brain separated from the rest of the body, one more line of defense against invaders such as germs, bacteria, and environmental toxins. I've always pictured this thin barrier like a bike helmet for our brain—an important layer of protection to minimize any negative impact. BDNF is also needed for neuroplasticity to take place—for the brain to change and improve. Because exercise helps to contribute to the production of BDNF, exercise helps facilitate development and learning. It also helps to protect against cognitive decline in adults. At this time, there are no supplements that directly impact BDNF. To produce BDNF, you must *move*.

Movement and exercise also release dopamine, a neurotransmitter that impacts our mood, energy, and motivation. When dopamine is low, there's a higher likelihood you'll experience brain fog, feel unmotivated, or feel sad. Dopamine is a part of the reward center in the brain, and it helps you anticipate pleasure, maintain hope, and feel motivated.[21] **The more you move and exercise, the more dopamine is released. That, in turn, teaches your brain to anticipate exercise and how it makes you feel. Frequent exercise and physical activity can help hardwire your brain to *like* exercise.**

When it comes to our young kids, movement and exercise occur naturally. If you've ever sat back and watched toddlers, you'll know what I mean. They are constantly on the go. Their brain and body crave movement to provide the stimulation and growth that contribute to their development. If adults moved as much and as often as toddlers, not only would we all be fit, but we'd also elevate our mood and cognition.

We hardly need to encourage our toddlers to move; on the contrary, we don't want to interfere with their movement impulses. Screen time detracts from what they'd naturally be doing—moving. A large study from the University of Calgary that looked at nearly 90,000 kids found that more than 75% of children younger than two years are exceeding screen time guidelines. Kids under age five are the fastest-growing users of digital media, engaging in screen time for 25% of their waking hours. Twenty-nine percent of babies younger than one watch an hour and a half of screens per day, and 64% of kids ages one to two years watch two hours per day.[22]

When interacting with toddlers, support a variety of movements. Find ways and places to jump, swim, pedal a trike, or climb. Different activities engage the brain and muscles in different ways, and, as they say, "variety is the spice of life."

Well-Being Activities for Infants and Toddlers

Sleep
- Create healthy sleep routines
- Bedtime routines shouldn't take too long and should be intended to prepare your child for rest: a warm bath, two short stories, a back rub, and a conversation about the day followed by hugs and kisses.

- Naps are critical. Kids this age still require a lot of sleep but often don't get it all overnight. Kids go through phases when they resist a nap, but that doesn't mean they are through with napping. If you stick to the routine, they'll often begin napping again. If they don't fall asleep during naptime, that's okay. Having quiet downtime on their own is still highly beneficial. It is a sensory break in their day and can help teach them how to entertain themselves. Keep technology out of this time. Have a rule that they need to stay in their room until it is time to get up, and have books or toys available so they can play quietly on their own.

Fuel
- In addition to fruits and veggies, growing and developing kids need protein, carbohydrates, and healthy fats to provide fuel for energy.
- Set a goal of providing protein at each meal and snack, five times per day.
- Protein snack ideas:
  - Protein smoothie
  - Nut butters: peanut, almond, cashew, or sunflower butter on anything—bread, bananas, rice cakes, crackers, celery sticks—or even a scoop straight from the jar
  - Collagen protein powder: Add plain or flavored collagen protein powder to cereal, smoothies, oatmeal, or muffins
  - Animal proteins: Use ground meat portioned in a muffin tin to make meatballs for an easy-to-chew animal protein option

Exercise
Remember, for toddlers, exercise is simply play and movement
- Run
- Jump
- Ride a scooter
- Climb
- Slide
- Swim
- Dance

- Hopscotch
- Play chase or tag
- Make obstacle courses of climbing over and under things
- Somersault down the hallway

Elementary School Students

Well-Being Milestones for Elementary School Students

Sleep recommendations by age:[23]
- Six to twelve years: 9–12 hours per day

Protein recommendations by age:[24]
- Five to eight years: 19 grams of protein per day
- Nine to thirteen years: 34 grams of protein per day

Screen time recommendations by age:[25]
- No more than one to two hours per day, keeping in mind that the time a child spends on a device is taking away from time being physically active, which the CDC refers to as screen time versus lean time

Even if your child is in elementary school, don't start reading here. Go back to the beginning of this chapter to learn about the three basic elements needed to support any brain: sleep, fuel, and exercise. I promise, you'll learn something you didn't already know.

As kids grow, it can be harder to control their sleep schedule and even the amount of movement and exercise they get. At the elementary age, you still often have a lot of influence over what foods they eat. Continue to be mindful of their sleep, fuel, and exercise so you can teach your kids the value of these important elements.

This generation of kids is gravitating toward more screen time, so working toward a healthy balance between screens and movement becomes increasingly important.

This is the perfect age to teach your kids how to support a healthy and fulfilled brain beyond the three basics of sleep, fuel, and exercise. The things they do—and then continue to do—influence which pathways in the brain become strong, fast, efficient, and easily accessible. While the topics in this section may at first sound like fluff, I assure you they are anything but. They are powerful tools for building a resilient brain. Gratitude, mindfulness, and understanding the importance of downtime are all practices that influence how much joy and fulfillment your child will experience.

The scientific journal *Frontiers in Psychology* published a study that concluded that expressing gratitude is a trigger for positive emotions, and the good news is you can cultivate or practice gratitude to bring more of those positive vibes into your child's life.[26] Like exercise, the more you practice gratitude, the more you strengthen the pathways to make it even easier. The Flow Research Collective podcast shared that the more you take time to practice gratitude, the more you notice and appreciate the little things and bring forth even more positive emotions.[27] If you talk, think, or write about gratitude, you'll start actively looking for things to be grateful for. You'll begin seeking more gratitude and joy. It's a positive feedback cycle—the more you do it, the more you see it.

Taking the time to notice and share what you are feeling grateful for is a simple but intentional act of purposefully activating happy feelings in your life. You can model this and create routines of gratitude with your kids that will benefit you both.

Whether you discuss what you're grateful for over dinner or in that quiet one-on-one time at bedtime, it's important to create a routine so your gratitude practice sticks. Hopefully, your child will carry on that routine, even when you're not guiding the activity.

It's easy to start a gratitude practice when you've had a great day and are in a good mood. It's much harder when you're exhausted or cranky or when stress levels are high. If the only thing you're grateful for that day is your bed to sleep in, or the sun in the sky, or the rain watering the plants outside, that's okay.

There's no wrong way to practice gratitude, but speaking out loud what you're grateful for engages the brain more than simply thinking the thoughts. Writing gratitude down is even more powerful.

Practicing gratitude is so powerful to the brain that leadership and corporate organizations include the concept in their workplace culture, as they have learned that a grateful leader results in more productive teams. The Wharton School of the University of Pennsylvania shares that "an active practice of gratitude increases neuron density and leads to higher emotional intelligence."[28] One way in which the business school integrates a gratitude practice into their culture is through Gratitude@Wharton, a platform for students dedicated to sharing gratitude for and with each other. With a slogan of "gratitude is the attitude," they strive to create an environment of finding ways to express gratitude daily. Who doesn't want that?

Your brain is a mass of neural pathways. In fact, remember that every neuron can connect with up to 1,000 other neurons each time it's fired and provide endless possibilities for your actions and reactions. The first time you do an action or have a thought is the first time that specific sequence of neurons is fired together. Then, each time you experience that same action or thought, that sequence fires again. The more you use that sequence, the stronger it becomes, making it easier to access.

Consider a jumping jack, a full-body activity that requires coordination and timing of both the upper and lower body. The first time you did a jumping jack as a child, it was most likely hard. You had to think about how to coordinate your arms and legs together in the correct direction at the correct time. But with practice, it became something you could do with ease. In fact, now you can most likely carry on a conversation or do mental math while doing jumping jacks. That's an example of a set pattern of neurons firing. You are able to execute an action or task without thought and with minimal effort.

Learning to read is another example. The first time you decode a word, sounding it out letter by letter, is the first time you fire that sequence of connections. The more you read that word, the easier it is to use those pathways, until a split-second glance at the word activates the pathways instantly and—voilà!—you have a sight word.

The same automaticity can happen with your thoughts. The first time someone bumps into you and you think, "you jerk," is the first time you fire that series of neurons. But over time, as you continue to respond the same way each time someone makes you mad, you strengthen the pathways that say, "when I get mad, I respond with 'you jerk!'" A strong pathway is easier to use. Do it enough and it becomes a habit, a pattern of neurons firing with very little effort.

You can begin to gain a little more control over the pathways you use and strengthen by becoming aware of how you feel and react. Realizing that when you get frustrated you say or think something unkind can help you pause and regroup. If you stop, take a few deep breaths, and think something different, it can become easier to access *other* pathways, such as those involved with empathy or gratitude.

Helping your child apply this concept is going to take some practice, guidance, and modeling from you. Remember that there is power in stating something out loud. Next time your child snaps at you in a rude tone of voice, instead of correcting them, or getting angry back, try pointing out what you are noticing and what it may indicate about how they're feeling. "I can hear in the tone of your voice and words that you're frustrated. I get it, everyone gets frustrated, and it isn't fun. I want to be able to help you, so let's work on this together." By kindly pointing out their tone and words, you are bringing awareness to how they are feeling. Next, you're showing them that it is okay to feel that way, and they're not alone. You're going to work with them to help reduce the frustration. By doing this over and over with your child, you are helping them build pathways to be aware of how they are feeling and acting and to communicate that information so that things can hopefully get better.

Mindfulness is the ability to be fully present in the moment and aware of your feelings, thoughts, and bodily sensations, which can lead, over time, to better control of your actions and reactions.[29] Mindfulness starts with being aware of how you feel, think, and react in various scenarios. To build this ability in your kids, continue to be a voice for them (and yes, this will definitely annoy them, but the goal is years from now they hear your voice in their head when they are upset and apply what you painstakingly worked to teach them). For example, when you realize that your child is tired and irritable, yet there is homework that still needs to be done, point out your observations and what you are going to do about it. "I can see by your mood and behavior that you're tired and crabby right now. That is going to make homework hard. We're going to take a few minutes together and use our muscles to help reset the brain, so we can be positive and productive." Or, next time you notice yourself feeling tired and crabby, share that information: "I'm really tired right now, so I won't tolerate the chaos very well this evening while I'm making dinner. I'm going to ask you to play outside while I'm cooking." Or, "I had a stressful day at work today, so I'm feeling really tense. I know some exercise right now or practicing gratitude may help me reset my brain to feel better." It will feel awkward in the beginning. Use Post-it notes to remind yourself until it feels more natural and becomes a habit to identify how you are feeling and what you can do about it, so you can help your kids do the same.

Our kids won't get there on their own, but with kind and gentle guidance, we can model mindfulness in ourselves and provide them with the words and awareness to help themselves: they might need quiet, food, rest, movement, or whatever you can think of that will help. Then talk about their experience after the fact. "I noticed that after you ate, you seemed much happier and more yourself. Did you notice that too?"

Helping kids identify what they're feeling and connect it to what they can do to *impact* how they're feeling just may provide a small sense of control in their lives.

Another important need for kids of all ages is downtime. The definition from Oxford Languages of *downtime* is a time of reduced activity or inactivity. And downtime is good for the brain. It helps support creativity, thought processing, balanced emotions, and even brainstorming. The key to downtime is that you're free from anything that requires effort, which can be mental effort or physical. It's a time of relaxation and can provide an opportunity for the mind to wander.

When presented with idle time, thoughts bounce from topic to topic and from the past to the present to the future. The default network is engaged, the pathways in the brain that are more active during passive times than active times. Remember that this *free-range thinking* time can help you to process events and experiences you've had and think about your life, and you just might do some amazing brainstorming.

In this era of technology, we've allowed our kids to spend more time with constant mental engagement, and less mental downtime engaging the default network pathways. At the beginning of the pandemic, it felt necessary so we could keep them engaged while we worked at home. None of us thought we'd be at home for nearly two years. But now, we need to purposefully shift those habits and routines. The second our kids aren't actively engaged in something specific, they reach for technology, and we need to redirect them so they're not gaming or scrolling aimlessly through videos on TikTok or YouTube.

Thoughts can sometimes be uncomfortable. Kids may think about a hard conversation they had with a friend or worry about an upcoming spelling test. But using technology to avoid those feelings sidesteps their free-range thinking and doesn't provide them with as much time to process their thoughts, feelings, and emotions.

When you limit technology use, be prepared to hear every parent's least favorite phrase: "I'm booooorrrreeed." Personally, I think boredom can be a good thing. During those times of boredom, kids become the most creative. They create forts out of cardboard boxes, tromp outside to catch fish in the creek, or get out a pen and paper to write a story. When you allow your kids the time and space to be alone with their thoughts, they often generate some of the most creative stories and deep-thinking questions you've ever seen.

It can be uncomfortable at first, so start by being aware of when downtime occurs for both you and your kids. Don't reach for your phone; instead, find something creative to do yourself and set a good example. Over time, downtime becomes quite comfortable.

To quote Tim Kreider, a writer and cartoonist, "Idleness is not just a vacation, an indulgence, or a vice. It is necessary. The space and quiet that idleness provides is a necessary condition."

Well-Being Activities for Elementary School Students

Practice gratitude

- Start by sharing what you're grateful for. Start small and simple. "Our dog, the warm weather today, you!" Then ask your child to share

something that makes them grateful. Challenge them to think of
something different each day.

- Create a gratitude routine around when and how you share your
  gratitude thoughts each day—over breakfast, driving in the car, at
  bedtime. Figure out what works for your family and make it a habit.
- Start a gratitude journal.
- Work together with your child to complete *The Gratitude and
  Affirmations Journal for Kids* by Jennifer Irwin. It's a great way to start
  a gratitude practice with your children. It guides both the child and
  the parent in starting this awareness and conversation. It also makes a
  great gift for kids.
- Notice how the more you practice gratitude, the more you'll notice
  yourself finding things to celebrate. Share these thoughts and
  observations with your kids to help them recognize and appreciate the
  positive impact of gratitude.

Instill mindfulness

- Identify the emotion you are experiencing, or your child may be
  experiencing in the moment or may soon face, then talk about
  the strategy you'll use to calm down and why. Later, when deeper
  communication is appropriate, talk about it again to reinforce it.
  - Model for your kids and start simple: "I'm feeling cold, so I'm
    going to grab a sweatshirt to wear." "I'm feeling thirsty, so I'm
    going to drink a glass of water."
- Tell your kids what you notice in them and, again, start simple.
  Connect an action to what you observe.
  - "I notice that your face is red, and you are sweaty. That tells
    me you're hot. Can I bring you a cold glass of water and cool
    washcloth to cool you down?"
- The moment of an upset isn't the time to discuss the observation and
  the action. In that moment, simply take gentle action. After they calm
  down, discuss your observations and actions.
  - "As your voice got louder and your words more angry, I realized
    you were upset and needed a quiet space to help you feel calm
    again."

- If you notice your child looking down, encourage them to choose something that will help spark good feelings—doing some exercise, planning something they love to do, spending time with a good friend, setting a goal, practicing gratitude, helping a friend.

Embrace downtime

Downtime can be active, as long as it isn't intense; it's simply a time of reduced activity or inactivity. A time when the mind isn't actively engaged in a task that requires thought or talking, and you do not need to exert effort. The mind is allowed to wander.

- Track downtime to increase your awareness for yourself and your kids! Set a goal of allowing space for downtime each day, even if it is only ten or fifteen minutes.
- Car time can be great downtime as long as devices aren't involved. Create a rule where phones aren't used in the car unless the drive is a certain distance.
- Go for a walk
- Use a meditation app (and by the way, it's okay and completely normal for your mind to wander as you begin to practice meditation; over time you will notice improvement in the ability to direct your thoughts and focus)
- Go fishing
- Color, draw, or paint
- Take a relaxing bath
- Sit quietly
- Snuggle the family pet
- Decorate cookies

Middle School and High School Students

Well-Being Milestones for Middle and High School Students

Sleep recommendations by age:[30]
- Thirteen to eighteen years: 8–10 hours

Protein recommendations by age:[31]

- Thirteen years: 34 grams of protein per day
- Girls fourteen to eighteen years: 46 grams of protein per day
- Boys fourteen to eighteen years: 52 grams of protein per day

Screen time recommendations by age:[32]

- No more than two hours a day of entertainment screen time (this does not include school or homework screen time)[33]

Part of development during the middle and high school years is a deepening sense of who you are and how you fit into your community and your world. At this age, kids navigate the world while experiencing surges of hormones and a heightening awareness of world events, and also navigating relationships with friends and family and beginning to engage in romantic relationships. They're filled with emotions and aspirations, and they don't always know how to handle these thoughts and feelings. Helping kids foster goals, a purpose in life, and connections through relationships can greatly add to their sense of self and community.

While there are many things we can do to bring joy and fulfillment to the brain, research has shown that finding a sense of passion and purpose in your life is one of the biggest contributing factors to leading a fulfilled life.

Nick Holton, a PhD in educational psychology who reviews manuscripts for the *Journal of Happiness Studies*, believes that people often sell themselves short, not striving to achieve more for fear they may fail, and as a result don't realize they're capable of so much more. In episode 42 of the "Flow Research Collective Podcast," Dr. Holton discusses the key to fulfillment in life is defining your passion and purpose.[34] He shares that finding a passion and purpose in life is not easy, but when this is accomplished it can help to push past that threshold of selling yourself short, so you have the drive and confidence to work toward achieving big things. Finding your passion, which is your energy for something, and your purpose, the driving reason behind your emotions, and pairing them together, provides you with both direction and fulfillment.

The good news is that your kids are allowed to have more than one passion and purpose in life, and it's okay if that changes and evolves over time as they, too, grow and evolve. The trick is to help them explore and foster the excitement and energy that naturally come from tapping into these feelings.

Dr. Holton recommends starting with curiosity: "Notice what naturally draws your kids' attention." What do they want to learn more about or do more of? Encourage that learning and exploration. Learning also brings happiness to the brain, so supporting ways for your kids to learn more about a topic or activity that excites them is positive in many ways. Ask questions, learn, and explore with them so that they can share what they love with you—that will strengthen the feeling of connection. Even if you don't love hockey, or whatever it is that they love, you *will* love the conversations and time spent with your child when you see their interest and enthusiasm! Not everything will lead to passion for an interest or activity, but they won't know if they don't try.

We've gotten to observe a passion and a hobby for Morgan, who loves to write. It's a passion that can keep her mentally engaged and stimulated for hours. She's been a storyteller from the time she could talk. When she was little, she made up elaborate stories about cats and mermaids and wrote them down as soon as she could form letters. Being an avid reader has inspired her to want to write and create her own stories even more. Whether she chooses to become a writer in her professional life or not, I have no doubt that she'll always be a writer to some degree. It captures her interest, and it challenges and excites her. When she gets an idea, we can go days when we barely see her while she's writing and illustrating images to go with her stories. Sparked with excitement and purpose, it drives her focus and energy in a way that makes her happy.

Finding a passion can be challenging, and what piques your interest at one point in life may not years later. Helping your kids explore different hobbies and activities will help them tap into various pursuits of interest and hopefully passion.

While the brain loves topics you are passionate about, the brain also loves a goal. In fact, I was surprised when I learned how much the brain loves goal setting, which I shouldn't have been, since my own brain *loves* setting goals. So much so that my husband makes fun of me for setting goals. I'll sign up with friends for a half marathon, hoping to spark some motivation to run more.

"Just go out and run," he'll say. "Why pay $60 and get a T-shirt when you can just run on your own?"

My answer: Because running on my own doesn't spark the same excitement as setting a goal with a friend, then reading about the course, filling out the form, paying money, and working to be half marathon–ready.

And now I know why. It turns out that when we set a goal, the brain releases dopamine. The brain truly does get excited about that goal—the passion that drives the decision to commit to something, and the anticipation of how good you'll feel or how proud you'll be when you accomplish your goal.

But, even though the brain loves setting a goal, it has a hard time staying on task to complete that goal. You've probably seen this in your own life. Can you think of goals you've set this year that you approached with full enthusiasm but that eventually fell by the wayside? The *New York Post* reported that by February 1, most people have abandoned their New Year's resolutions.[35] Why is this?

The brain experiences a surge of dopamine, energy, and excitement when you set a goal, but dopamine doesn't stay active in the brain for long, which means that excitement and anticipation wane. This is when the hard work comes in to achieve a goal. You have to dig deep, utilize your energy and effort, and tap into those higher-level brain pathways to override your habits and patterns—all things that aren't easy to do.

So how do you keep the brain happy and energized to help you fulfill that goal, which the brain *really* loves? Break up the goal into smaller parts—into mini-goals that are achievable in a shorter amount of time. Each mini-goal is still a goal that will excite the brain, and achieving that goal will help re-engage the excitement and energy needed for the next step.

For years, my son had the goal to play for a travel hockey team. Even though we live in the South, we have an excellent hockey development program that has grown and become far more competitive over the years. While jumping up a big level in play felt overwhelming, my husband helped Drew break it up into some mini-goals. Step-by-step, Drew focused on what he needed to accomplish: lifting the puck when shooting; learning to aim for a specific spot in the net and not the center mass of the goalie; developing a powerful wrist shot for when he didn't have as much time and space on the ice to line things up perfectly. For each of those tasks, my husband explained what the goal was and what Drew needed to do in practice to get there. Drew got excited because he could imagine the impact it would have on his game. Then he'd spend hours in the driveway practicing (and denting the garage doors in the process). The next game would come around, and when Drew could successfully put what he practiced into action, that achievement would double-down his focus and determination to achieve the next goal.

As parents, we can help make our child's goal a reality by showing them how to break it down into the necessary steps and by providing structure and encouragement along the way. Each goal achieved will only provide more motivation and ability to achieve the next!

Supporting a resilient brain in teens also means fostering good friendships. Good social relationships are the most consistent predictor of a happy life.[36] Study after study confirms it. Meaningful connections and relationships are critical in our lives, which is why the past couple of years have been so hard on our teens. They had fewer opportunities to interact and to practice and learn from social interactions. Social relationships support their feelings of being relevant, loved, and a part of something. While they'll always need love and support from you, at this age they have a larger need for outside validation and connection. They need to form their own peer circles.

Joy comes from both *being* a good friend and *having* good friends—being there to support a friend who needs a sympathetic ear and having a friend to support them in times of frustration or upset. They need to know that they're surrounded by love and friendship, so when they need to talk to someone, dream about the future, or share a laugh, they have their group of people who support them.

Well-Being Activities for Middle School and High School Students

Everything we've discussed throughout this book is focused on supporting overall well-being. Foundational development in core muscles, coordination, sensory perception, timing, and fine motor skills build the neural pathways that lead to attention, memory, inhibitory control, and cognitive flexibility, which lead to a more resilient brain with improved awareness and control over mood and behaviors. Combining the exercises throughout the book will help to exercise and improve those pathways. Then, being mindful about the additional activities and exercises shared here can help to create a more balanced life.

In addition to the activities shared earlier in this chapter, having a focus on these areas will contribute to your teen's overall well-being:

- Find a passion and purpose
  - Volunteer
  - Try new hobbies until one creates excitement and a desire to learn and do more
  - Encourage your teen to build or create something on their own—cook, bake, build, write, sing, dance, sew, craft—anything that is created from scratch can provide a sense of accomplishment and pride
- Practice goal setting
  - Work together with your teens and create goals in several categories: school, friendships, home, health, fitness, sports, and so on
  - Set a big goal, then work together to break the goal into smaller sections.
  - Write the goals down and include dates, then keep them someplace as a visual reminder to help stay on track for achieving them.
- Help your child find community and connections through in-person interactions (not just gaming online together)
- Create opportunities for multiple communities
  - While having close and meaningful connections and relationships has been shown to be an important contributor to feelings of well-being, there is also joy and value in seeing familiar faces and feeling welcome in various groups. Examples can include a religious youth

group, a weekly gym class, a sports team, or a group with a similar interest as your child.

Signs That Indicate Improvement

When your child increases in maturity and it's reflected in their emotional well-being, it doesn't mean they'll be happy all the time. But they will be more adept at handling their moods and emotions and will know what to do to continue to stay in control and be productive. This is a lifelong learning curve that we parents can support, learn, and apply to ourselves too. Our actions impact our mood—it's a matter of cause and effect. But the impact isn't always immediately evident, which can make it difficult to understand and apply.

While each child is different, watch for the subtle clues that your child feels fulfilled, connected, and content. Some young kids will skip or sing when they're happy; older kids may engage more in conversation and activities at home, be more willing to engage with people they don't know as well, or try doing something new. Be aware if you see a shift in your child. Engaging these techniques will help their brain feel more rested and positive as they practice gratitude, purpose, and connection.

Maturity and development in well-being will come with improved awareness and action. When you notice your child adjusting what they are doing in order to support their productivity, energy, and mood, you'll know that self-awareness and the executive functions needed to make good decisions are kicking in to support their well-being.

EPILOGUE

· · · ·

CREATING YOUR ACTION PLAN

opefully, reading this book provided you with some new insights, ideas, and inspiration. While it isn't realistic to work all the activities into each day, mapping out a purposeful plan to use as a guide can help you create a positive routine of brain engagement and strengthening.

I encourage you to engage your child in this process as much as possible if developmentally appropriate for them (I wouldn't ask a two-year-old which activities they'd want to do). For a young child, you could present them with two options: "We're going to do a brain exercise now, would you like to do X or Y today?" This provides your child with an element of control, while still accomplishing what is needed to support their development.

Parents often ask me how they should talk to their child about their child's challenges, or the exercises and activities they're doing to help them. If your child has the developmental ability to be aware of some of their challenges and how they are impacting them, I would discuss this with your child before starting the exercises. I always encourage honesty, but with kindness and hope. I like to explain to both kids and adults that the brain is complex, and we all have areas that would benefit from exercise. We all also have areas of strengths, and areas that could be improved, and sometimes the areas that could be improved can make life really tough. Having an area of the brain that would benefit from strengthening or improvement does not mean they're not an awesome kid, or smart, or strong. It means that we have an opportunity to work to make a difference in something that is hard. "I know how hard you work at school to listen and to not interrupt or disrupt, and I understand how hard that is for you. We have a chance to do some special activities to exercise the part of your brain that supports attention and impulse control so we can help that be easier for you. I'd love my attention to be better too, let's work on this together."

If your child is younger in their development, I would keep it simple: "Time to do exercises to help make our brains stronger!"

Each chapter in the book contains important elements that contribute to overall development and well-being, so your action plan should include elements from each chapter. Every child will also have areas of higher priority where more symptoms and struggles are present. For those areas, you'll have a larger weekly emphasis on those activities.

- Regardless of your child's current age, review the milestone activities in each chapter for all three age groups and check off the milestones your child has already achieved.
- Identify if you have a high-priority area. If your child has multiple high priorities (which is often the case), proceed through the book in order, starting with coordination development as your initial high priority, then shifting to sensory development, fine motor development, and so on.
- Highlight the activities from each chapter you think would work well for your child, reviewing activities for all three age groups. If age appropriate, have your child participate in helping to identify activities they would want to do.
- Create a plan for the best time of day or time during the week to do each activity. For example, as a part of your bedtime routine, while in the car, or on the weekend.

For each of the following categories, create a list of starting activities, then fill in the calendar using a variety of activities from each category to create your monthly plan. At the end of each month you can update your calendar to continue to work through a wide variety of activities.

Developmental categories:

- Coordination
- Sensory
- Fine motor
- Attention
- Relationships
- Learning
- Upsets
- Anxiety
- Well-being

Opportunities to incorporate developmental activities:

- Morning routine
- After school
- Homework routine
- After dinner
- Bedtime
- Weekend
- In the car

Remember, whenever possible, to layer stimulation and activities to engage more pathways in the brain to fire at the same time. To layer, it can be helpful to start with a foundational exercise. Then, once your child has mastered that exercise, add another element to it. For example, you can have your child do the exercise while talking about their day, or do the exercise with music while playing a memory game.

Applying the suggestions and activities in this book will take a plan and effort, and working with your own child can be challenging, but I can't think of a more important reason to put in the work than helping your child thrive.

The brain is at the core of all we do—influencing our thoughts, emotions, learning, and interactions with the world. When the brain is optimized, there is a larger opportunity to truly be present and engaged with the environment and to get the most out of every experience. The world's top athletes understand the importance of exercising the brain to maximize all they do to keep them at the top of their game. You have that same opportunity to optimize the abilities and performance of your child's brain—at any age. The science of neuroplasticity has shown us that the brain can change, and these changes can impact quality of life. Working together with your child to understand how to strengthen and engage their brain may be one of the best gifts you can provide to them, impacting their lives not just today but every day going forward.

We can't undo the past, but we can learn, grow, and optimize the future for our kids by applying what we've learned from a tumultuous time. The prolonged pandemic response reinforced the importance of sensory exposure, movement, relationships, and the need to support a healthy, efficient, and optimized brain to live an optimized life.

ACKNOWLEDGMENTS

I am so appreciative of the people in my life who have helped shape me, as well as this project. While my name is credited as the author, every thought and word has been influenced by my life experiences and the insight and support of those around me. This is my thank-you card to the countless people who have impacted me in a meaningful way.

Thank you to Doug, my true partner in every sense of the word. You listen often, redirect my energy sometimes, and love always.

To my parents, I am who I am because of you, and for that I am forever grateful. You gave me the encouragement, love, and support to chase my dreams and demonstrated the value of hard work and family.

To Morgan and Drew who keep every day an adventure and provide so much meaning and joy in my life.

To my sisters who are my constants, who roll their eyes while still encouraging me, there can never be enough sister trips and adventures.

To the girlfriends in my life both near and far, who celebrate life with me, lift me up when I'm questioning myself, and share so many moments of laughter and tambourines—the perfect balance to the daily grind of life.

To all the true book professionals that guided this novice through the process of making a lifelong dream a reality. My editor, Daniela Rapp, my book coach, Nancy Erickson, and my agent, Carol Mann, as well as the entire editing team at Mayo Clinic Press, who directed this process to polish my work, while staying true to my voice.

To the entire Brain Balance community. After 15 years I am still learning. I'm so thankful for the opportunities I've had to learn, work hard, grow, collaborate, and contribute to something that has touched the lives of tens of thousands of people. To see or hear from a former student or family a decade later and learn about the lasting impact of our work reignites my joy and passion to do more every time.

To the photographer who said, "The babies are different" and sparked the energy in me to put pen to paper and try and help in some small way the millions of kids and families struggling.

To the readers for whom my hope is that you find some words or ideas within these pages that will help you impact the lives of those you love.

Thank you.

—*Rebecca*

NOTES

Introduction

1. Melinda Wenner Moyer, "The COVID Generation: How Is the Pandemic Affecting Kids' Brains?" *Nature* 601 (January 12, 2022), https://www.nature.com/articles/d41586-022-00027-4.
2. Megan Kuhfeld, James Soland, and Karyn Lewis, "Test Score Patterns across Three COVID-19-Impacted School Years," *Educational Researcher* 7, no. 51 (June 30, 2022): 521.
3. David K. Li, "Youth Suicide Attempts Soared during Pandemic," NBC News, June 11, 2021, http://www.nbcnews.com/news/us-news/youth-suicide-attempts-soared-during-pandemic-cdc-report-says-n1270463.
4. Sarah Mervosh and Ashley Wu, "Math Scores Fell in Nearly Every State and Reading Dipped on National Exam," *New York Times*, October 24, 2022, http://www.nytimes.com/2022/10/24/us/math-reading-scores-pandemic.html.
5. Adrienne L. Tierney and Charles A. Nelson III, "Brain Development and the Role of Experience in the Early Years," *Zero Three* 30, no. 2 (November 1, 2009): 9–13.
6. Tierney and Nelson, "Brain Development."
7. Weiyan Yin, Tengfei Li, Peter J. Mucha, Jessica R. Cohen, Hongtu Zhu, Ziliang Li, and Weili Lin, "Altered Neural Flexibility in Children with Attention-Deficit/Hyperactivity Disorder," *Molecular Psychiatry* 27 (July 22, 2022): 4673–4679.
8. Tierney and Nelson, "Brain Development."
9. Lawrence Green, "Closing the Chasm between Research and Practice: Evidence of and for Change," *Health Promotion Journal of Australia* 25, no. 1 (April 2014): 25–29, DOI: 10.1071/HE13101.

Chapter 1

1. Adrienne L. Tierney and Charles A. Nelson III, "Brain Development and the Role of Experience in the Early Years," *Zero Three* 30, no. 2 (November 1, 2009): 9–13.
2. The Brain Balance Multi-Domain Developmental Survey is available to view in the published study: Rebecca Jackson and Josh Jordan, "Measurement Properties of the Brain Balance® Multidomain Developmental Survey: Validated Factor Structure, Internal Reliability, and Measurement Invariance," *Current Psychology* (2023), https://doi.org/10.1007/s12144-023-04248-2.
3. Kirstin Macdonald, Nikki Milne, Robin Orr, and Rodney Pope, "Relationships between Motor Proficiency and Academic Performance in Mathematics and Reading in School-Aged Children and Adolescents: A Systematic Review," *International Journal*

of Environmental Research and Public Health 15, no. 8 (July 28, 2018): 1603, DOI: 10.1038/d41586-022-00027-4.

4. Jan P. Piek and Murray J. Dyck, "Sensory-Motor Deficits in Children with Developmental Coordination Disorder, Attention Deficit Hyperactivity Disorder and Autistic Disorder," *Human Movement Science* 23, no. 3–4 (2004): 475–488.

5. Melinda Wenner Moyer, "The COVID Generation: How Is the Pandemic Affecting Kids' Brains?" *Nature* 601, no. 7892 (January 2022): 180–183.

6. Macdonald et al., "Relationships between Motor Proficiency and Academic Performance."

7. Moyer, "The COVID Generation."

8. Moyer, "The COVID Generation"; Macdonald et al., "Relationships between Motor Proficiency and Academic Performance"; Svend Sparre Geertsen, Richard Thomas, Malte Neijst Larsen, Ida Marie Dahn, Josefine Needham Andersen, Matilde Krause-Jensen, Claus Malta Nielsen, Vibeke Korup, et al., "Motor Skills and Exercise Capacity Are Associated with Objective Measures of Cognitive Functions and Academic Performance in Preadolescent Children," *PloS One* 11, no. 8 (2016): e0161960; Lauren E. Miller, Jeffrey D. Burke, Eva Troyb, Kelley Knoch, Lauren E. Herlihy, and Deborah A. Fein, "Preschool Predictors of School-Age Academic Achievement in Autism Spectrum Disorder," *Clinical Neuropsychologist* 31, no. 2 (2017): 382–403.

9. Matt Richtel, "Children's Screen Time Has Soared in the Pandemic, Alarming Parents and Researchers," *New York Times*, January 16, 2021, http://nytimes.com/2021/01/16/health/covid-kids-tech-use.html.

10. Fayiqa Ahamed Bahkir and Srinivasan Subramanian Grandee, "Impact of the COVID-19 Lockdown on Digital Device-Related Ocular Health," *Indian Journal of Ophthalmology* 68, no. 11 (November 2020): 2378.

11. Richtel, "Children's Screen Time Has Soared in the Pandemic, Alarming Parents and Researchers."

12. Joseph H. Arguinchona and Prasanna Tadi, "Neuroanatomy, Reticular Activating System," *StatPearls* (2022, updated July 25, 2022), https://ncbi.nlm.nih.gov/books/NBK549835/.

13. "CDC's Developmental Milestones," Centers for Disease Control and Prevention, last modified December 29, 2022, https://www.cdc.gov/ncbddd/actearly/milestones/index.html.

14. Bahkir and Grandee, "Impact of the COVID-19 Lockdown on Digital Device-Related Ocular Health"; "CDC's Developmental Milestones."

15. Bahkir and Grandee, "Impact of the COVID-19 Lockdown on Digital Device-Related Ocular Health."

16. Bahkir and Grandee, "Impact of the COVID-19 Lockdown on Digital Device-Related Ocular Health."

17. "How Physical Skills Develop, Age by Age," Scholastic (April 2019), accessed January 29, 2023, https://www.scholastic.com/parents/family-life/social-emotional-learning/development-milestones/how-physical-skills-develop-age-age.html.

18. "How Physical Skills Develop, Age by Age."

19. Bahkir and Grandee, "Impact of the COVID-19 Lockdown on Digital Device-Related Ocular Health."

20. Bahkir and Grandee, "Impact of the COVID-19 Lockdown on Digital Device-Related Ocular Health."
21. Bahkir and Grandee, "Impact of the COVID-19 Lockdown on Digital Device-Related Ocular Health."
22. Bahkir and Grandee, "Impact of the COVID-19 Lockdown on Digital Device-Related Ocular Health."
23. Bahkir and Grandee, "Impact of the COVID-19 Lockdown on Digital Device-Related Ocular Health."
24. Bahkir and Grandee, "Impact of the COVID-19 Lockdown on Digital Device-Related Ocular Health."
25. "Presidential Youth Fitness Program," U.S. Department of Health and Human Services, accessed January 29, 2023, https://health.gov/our-work/nutrition-physical-activity/presidents-council/programs-awards/presidential-youth-fitness-program.
26. "Presidential Youth Fitness Program." Bold is my addition.
27. "Presidential Youth Fitness Program."
28. "What Is Bone-Strengthening Exercise?" Healthcarefix, accessed January 29, 2023, https://healthcarefix.com/what-is-bone-strengthening-exercise/.
29. "Developing into Teenage Years," OT for Kids, accessed March 16, 2023, https://www.otforkids.co.uk/problems-we-help/delayed-milestones/developing-into-teenage-years-10-to-15-years.php.
30. Jean M. Twenge and W. Keith Campbell, "Associations between Screen Time and Lower Psychological Well-Being among Children and Adolescents: Evidence from a Population-Based Study," *Preventive Medicine Reports* 12 (October 18, 2018): 271–283, DOI: 10.1016/j.pmedr.2018.10.003.

Chapter 2

1. Matthew T. Birnie and Tallie Z. Baram, "Principles of Emotional Brain Circuit Maturation," *Science* 376, no. 6597 (June 2, 2022): 1055–1056, DOI: 10.1126/science.abn4016.
2. "Cognition," Wikipedia, accessed January 29, 2023, https://en.wikipedia.org/wiki/Cognition.
3. Rebecca Jackson and Conor J. Wild, "Effect of the Brain Balance Program® on Cognitive Performance in Children and Adolescents with Developmental and Attentional Issues," *Journal of Advances in Medicine and Medical Research* 33, no. 6 (March 2021): 27–41.
4. "Your Brain at Work: The Reticular Activating System (RAS) and Your Goals and Behaviour," lifexchangessolutions.com, accessed January 29, 2023, https://lifexchangesolutions.com/reticular-activating-system/.
5. "Sensory Processing Issues after Traumatic Events," Solstice Residential Treatment Center, July 22, 2021, https://solsticertc.com/sensory-processing-issues-after-traumatic-events/#:~:text=Many%20people%20become%20hypervigilant%20to,of%20safety%20in%20the%20present.
6. David R. Moore, Justin A. Cowan, Alison Riley, Mark Edmondson-Jones, and Melanie A. Ferguson, "Development of Auditory Processing in 6- to 11-Year-Old Children," *Ear and Hearing* 32, no 3. (May–June 2011): 269–285, DOI: 10.1097/AUD.0b013e318201c468.

7. Jewel E. Crasta, Emily Salzinger, Mei-Heng Lin, William J. Gavin, and Patricia L. Davies, "Sensory Processing and Attention Profiles among Children with Sensory Processing Disorders and Autism Spectrum Disorders," *Frontiers in Integrative Neuroscience* 14, no. 22 (May 5, 2020), DOI: 10.3389/fnint.2020.00022.

8. Gina Shaw, "The Truth about Sensory Processing Disorder," WebMD, June 21, 2012, accessed January 29, 2023, https://www.webmd.com/children/features/the-truth-about -sensory-processing-disorder.

9. "Resources by Age," Pathways, 2023, accessed January 29, 2023, https://pathways.org /growth-development/0-3-months/milestones/.

10. "Resources by Age."

11. "Resources by Age."

12. "Resources by Age."

13. "Resources by Age."

14. Elise Hancock, "The Handy Guide to Touch," *Johns Hopkins Magazine*, electronic edition (April 1995), accessed May 3, 2022, https://pages.jh.edu/jhumag/495web/touch .html.

15. "Tactile Sensitivity," scienceworld.ca, June 30, 2020, https://www.scienceworld.ca /resource/tactile-sensitivity/.

16. "Sensory/Social Skills: 2 to 12 Years," Children's Hospital of Richmond at Virginia Commonwealth University, 2023, accessed January 29, 2023, https://www.chrichmond .org/services/therapy-services/developmental-milestones/sensorysocial-skills-2-to-12 -years.

17. Silje Steinsbekk, Arielle Bonneville-Roussy, Alison Fildes, Clare H. Llewellyn, and Lars Wichstrøm, "Child and Parent Predictors of Picky Eating from Preschool to School Age," *International Journal of Behavioral and Nutrition and Physical Activity* 14, no. 87 (July 6, 2017), DOI: 10.1186/s12966-017-0542-7.

18. David Robson, "Interoception: The Hidden Sense That Shapes Well-Being," *The Guardian*, August 15, 2021, https://www.theguardian.com/science/2021/aug/15/the -hidden-sense-shaping-your-wellbeing-interoception#:~:text=Scientists%20have%20 shown%20that%20our,such%20as%20anxiety%20and%20depression.

19. Mark Beech, "COVID-19 Pushes Up Internet Use 70% and Streaming More than 12%, First Figures Reveal," *Forbes*, March 26, 2020, https://www.forbes.com/sites/mark beech/2020/03/25/covid-19-pushes-up-internet-use-70-streaming-more-than-12-first -figures-reveal/?sh=4b7e36be3104.

20. Beech, "COVID-19 Pushes Up Internet Use 70% and Streaming More than 12%, First Figures Reveal."

21. David K. Li, "Youth Suicide Attempts Soared during Pandemic, CDC Report Says," NBC News, June 11, 2021, https://www.nbcnews.com/news/us-news/youth-suicide -attempts-soared-during-pandemic-cdc-report-says-n1270463.

22. Apurvakumar Pandya and Pragya Lodha, "Social Connectedness, Excessive Screen Time during COVID-19 and Mental Health: A Review of Current Evidence," *Frontiers in Human Dynamics* 3 (July 22, 2021): 45, DOI: 10.3389/fhumd.2021.684137.

23. Amishi P. Jha, *Peak Mind: Find Your Focus, Own Your Attention, Invest 12 Minutes a Day* (London: Hachette, 2021).

Chapter 3

1. Matt Richtel, "Children's Screen Time Has Soared in the Pandemic, Alarming Parents and Researchers," *New York Times*, January 16, 2021, https://www.nytimes.com/2021/01/16/health/covid-kids-tech-use.html.

2. Gerald Giesbrecht, Catherine Lebel, Cindy-Lee Dennis, Suzanne C. Tough, Sheila McDonald, and Lianne Tomfohr-Madsen, "Increased Risk for Developmental Delay among Babies Born during the Pandemic" (pre-print), PsyArXiv, February 3, 2022, https://psyarxiv.com/j7kcn/.

3. "Infant Vision: Birth to 24 Months of Age," American Optometric Association, accessed January 29, 2023, https://www.aoa.org/healthy-eyes/eye-health-for-life/infant-vision?sso=y#:~:text=By%20eight%20weeks%2C%20babies%20begin,This%20is%20usually%20normal.

4. Ueli Suter and Rudolf Martini, "Myelination," in *Peripheral Neuropathy*, 4th ed., edited by Peter J. Dyck and P. K. Thomas (Philadelphia: W.B. Saunders, 2005), 411–431, DOI: 10.1016/B978-0-7216-9491-7.50022-3.

5. "CDC's Developmental Milestones," Centers for Disease Control and Prevention, last modified December 29, 2022, https://www.cdc.gov/ncbddd/actearly/milestones/index.html.

6. Russel Lazarus, "Vision Development and Milestones," Optometrists Network, May 4, 2020, https://www.optometrists.org/childrens-vision/guide-to-visual-development/guide-to-vision-development/; Beatriz Luna, Katerina Velanova, and Charles F. Geier, "Development of Eye-Movement Control," *Brain and Cognition* 68, no. 3 (December 2008): 293–308, DOI: 10.1016/j.bandc.2008.08.019; Dorian Smith-Garcia, "All about Baby Vision Development," HealthLine, September 29, 2020, https://www.healthline.com/health/baby/baby-vision.

7. Sally Goddard, *Reflexes, Learning and Behavior: A Window into the Child's Mind: A Non-Invasive Approach to Solving Learning and Behavior Problems* (Eugene, OR: Fern Ridge Press, 2002).

8. "Child Development Charts," KidSense, accessed January 29, 2023, https://childdevelopment.com.au/resources/child-development-charts/.

9. Lazarus, "Vision Development and Milestones"; Luna et al., "Development of Eye-Movement Control."

10. Lazarus, "Vision Development and Milestones."

11. Lazarus, "Vision Development and Milestones."

12. Xiujuan Zhang, Stephanie S. L. Cheung, Hei-Nga Chan, Yuzhou Zhang, Yu Meng Wang, Benjamin H. Yip, Ka Wai Kam, et al., "Myopia Incidence and Lifestyle Changes among School Children during the COVID-19 Pandemic: A Population-Based Prospective Study," *British Journal of Ophthalmology* 106, no. 12 (November 22, 2022): 1772–1778.

13. Maria Camila Cortés-Albornoz, Sofia Ramírez-Guerrero, William Rojas-Carabali, Alejandra de-la-Torre, and Claudia Talero-Gutiérrez, "Effects of Remote Learning during the COVID-19 Lockdown on Children's Visual Health: A Systematic Review," *BMJ Open* 12, no. 8 (2022): e062388, DOI: 10.1136/bmjopen-2022-062388.

Chapter 4

1. Jack Hollingdale, Nicoletta Adamo, and Kevin Tierney, "Impact of COVID-19 for People Living and Working with ADHD: A Brief Review of the Literature," *AIMS Public Health* 8, no. 4 (August 23, 2021): 581, DOI: 10.3934/publichealth.2021047.

2. Tessa Peasgood, Anupam Bhardwaj, Katie Biggs, John E. Brazier, David Coghill, Cindy L. Cooper, David Daley, et al., "The Impact of ADHD on the Health and Well-Being of ADHD Children and Their Siblings," *European Child and Adolescent Psychiatry* 25, no. 11 (April 1, 2016): 1217–1231, DOI: 10.1007/s00787-016-0841-6.

3. Anna-Mariya Kirova, Caroline Kelberman, Barbara Storch, Maura DiSalvo, K. Yvonne Woodworth, Stephen V. Faraone, and Joseph Biederman, "Are Subsyndromal Manifestations of Attention Deficit Hyperactivity Disorder Morbid in Children? A Systematic Qualitative Review of the Literature with Meta-Analysis," *Psychiatry Research* 274 (April 2019): 75–90, DOI: 10.1016/j.psychres.2019.02.003.

4. Orsolya Király, Marc N. Potenza, Dan J. Stein, Daniel L. King, David C. Hodgis, John B. Saunders, Mark D. Griffiths, et al., "Preventing Problematic Internet Use during the COVID-19 Pandemic: Consensus Guidance," *Comprehensive Psychiatry* 100 (July 2020): 152–180.

5. "ADHD Symptoms Unmasked by the Pandemic: Diagnoses Spike among Adults, Children," ADDitude, March 31, 2021, https://www.additudemag.com/adhd-symptoms -diagnosed-treated-in-pandemic/.

6. Hollingdale et al., "Impact of COVID-19 for People Living and Working with ADHD."

7. Randy L. Buckner, "The Brain's Default Network: Origins and Implications for the Study of Psychosis," *Dialogues in Clinical Neuroscience* 15, no. 3 (2013): 351–358.

8. Amishi P. Jha, *Peak Mind: Find Your Focus, Own Your Attention, Invest 12 Minutes a Day* (London: Hachette, 2021).

9. "Know Your Brain: Default Mode Network," Neuroscientifically Challenged, accessed January 29, 2023, https://neuroscientificallychallenged.com/posts/know-your-brain -default-mode-network.

10. Anna MacKay-Brandt, "Focused Attention," in *Encyclopedia of Clinical Neuropsychology*, edited by J. S. Kreutzer, J. DeLuca, and B. Caplan (New York: Springer, 2011), 1066–1067, DOI: 10.1007/978-0-387-79948-3_1303.

11. MacKay-Brandt, "Focused Attention."

12. Colleen Killingsworth, "Parents Sue Fortnite Creator for 'Knowingly' Making an 'Addictive Game,' Comparing It to Drug," Fox TV Stations, October 7, 2019, accessed January 23, 2023, https://www.fox10phoenix.com/news/parents-sue-fortnite-creator -for-knowingly-making-an-addictive-game-comparing-it-to-drug.

13. Chris Pennington, "We Are Hardwired to Resist Change," Emerson Human Capital Consulting, April 3, 2018, https://www.emersonhc.com/change-management/people -hard-wired-resist-change.

14. Jha, *Peak Mind.*

15. Pennington, "We Are Hardwired to Resist Change."

16. Jan P. Piek and Murray J. Dyck, "Sensory-Motor Deficits in Children with Developmental Coordination Disorder, Attention Deficit Hyperactivity Disorder and Autistic Disorder," *Human Movement Science* 23, no. 3–4 (2004): 475–488.

17. "CDC's Developmental Milestones," Centers for Disease Control and Prevention, last modified December 29, 2022, https://www.cdc.gov/ncbddd/actearly/milestones/index .html.

18. "CDC's Developmental Milestones."

19. "Important Developmental Milestones: A Timeline for Typical Development," Brain Balance, accessed January 29, 2023, https://www.brainbalancecenters.com/blog /important-developmental-milestones-timeline-typical-development.

20. Myra Taylor, Stephen Houghton, and Elaine Chapman, "Primitive Reflexes and Attention-Deficit/Hyperactivity Disorder: Developmental Origins of Classroom Dysfunction," *International Journal of Special Education* 19, no. 1 (2004): 23–37.

21. Taylor et al., "Primitive Reflexes and Attention-Deficit/Hyperactivity Disorder."

22. Taylor et al., "Primitive Reflexes and Attention-Deficit/Hyperactivity Disorder."

23. Sally Goddard, *Reflexes, Learning and Behavior: A Window into the Child's Mind: A Non-Invasive Approach to Solving Learning and Behavior Problems* (Eugene, OR: Fern Ridge Press, 2002).

24. Ewa Z. Gieysztor, Anna M. Choińska, and Małgorzata Paprocka-Borowicz, "Persistence of Primitive Reflexes and Associated Motor Problems in Healthy Preschool Children," *Archives of Medical Science* 14, no. 1 (2018): 167.

25. Piek and Dyck, "Sensory-Motor Deficits in Children with Developmental Coordination Disorder, Attention Deficit Hyperactivity Disorder and Autistic Disorder."

26. "CDC's Developmental Milestones."

27. "CDC's Developmental Milestones."

28. "CDC's Developmental Milestones."

29. "CDC's Developmental Milestones."

30. Taylor et al., "Primitive Reflexes and Attention-Deficit/Hyperactivity Disorder."

31. Taylor et al., "Primitive Reflexes and Attention-Deficit/Hyperactivity Disorder."

32. Martin H. Teicher, Elizabeth Bolger, Poopak Hafezi, Laura C. Hernandez Garcia, Cynthia E. McGreenery, Leslie Weiser, Kyoko Ohashi, and Alaptagin Khan, "Open Assessment of the Therapeutic and Rate-Dependent Effects of Brain Balance Center® and Interactive Metronome® Exercises on Children with Attention Deficit Hyperactivity Disorder," *Psychiatry Research* 319 (2023), DOI: 10.1016/j.psychres .2022.114973.

33. John J. Ratey, *Spark: The Revolutionary New Science of Exercise and the Brain* (London: Hachette, 2008).

34. "Short-Term Exercise Equals Big-Time Brain Boost: Even a One-Time, Brief Burst of Exercise Can Improve Focus, Problem-Solving," ScienceDaily, December 21, 2017, https://www.sciencedaily.com/releases/2017/12/171221122543.htm.

35. "Short-Term Exercise Equals Big-Time Brain Boost."

36. "CDC's Developmental Milestones."

37. "CDC's Developmental Milestones."

38. Jha, *Peak Mind.*

39. Jha, *Peak Mind.*

40. Catherine J. Norris, Daniel Creem, Reuben Hendler, and Hedy Kober, "Brief Mindfulness Meditation Improves Attention in Novices: Evidence from Erps and

Moderation by Neuroticism," *Frontiers in Human Neuroscience* 12 (August 6, 2018): 315.

41. Wikipedia, "Mindfulness," accessed March 15, 2023, https://en.wikipedia.org/wiki /Mindfulness.

42. Flow Research Collective, "Zen & Flow: How Zen Masters Tap into Flow w/ Henry Shukman," August 4, 2022, https://www.flowresearchcollective.com/radio/zen-flow -how-zen-masters-tap-into-flow.

43. A. Ganguly, S. M. Hulke, R. Bharshanakar, R. Parashar, S. Wakode, "Effect of Meditation on Autonomic Function in Healthy Individuals: A Longitudinal Study," *Journal of Family Medicine and Primary Care* 9, no. 8 (August 2020): 3944–3948, DOI: 10.4103/jfmpc.jfmpc_460_20. PMID: 33110791; PMCID: PMC7586536.

44. Emma Seppälä, "How Meditation Benefits CEOs," *Harvard Business Review*, December 14, 2015, https://hbr.org/2015/12/how-meditation-benefits-ceos.

Chapter 5

1. Jean M. Twenge, Jonathan Haidt, Andrew B. Blake, Cooper McAllister, Hannah Lemon, and Astrid Le Roy, "Worldwide Increases in Adolescent Loneliness," *Journal of Adolescence* 93 (December 2021): 257–269.

2. Amarica Rafanelli, "Growing Up in a Pandemic: How Covid Is Affecting Children's Development," Direct Relief, January 19, 2021, https://www.directrelief.org/2021/01 /growing-up-in-the-midst-of-a-pandemic-how-covid-is-affecting-childrens-development/.

3. Melinda Wenner Moyer, "The COVID Generation: How Is the Pandemic Affecting Kids' Brains?" *Nature*, January 12, 2022, https://www.nature.com/articles/d41586 -022-00027-4.

4. Liz Mineo, "Good Genes Are Nice, but Joy Is Better," *Harvard Gazette*, April 11, 2017, accessed January 23, 2023, https://news.harvard.edu/gazette/story/2017/04/over-nearly -80-years-harvard-study-has-been-showing-how-to-live-a-healthy-and-happy-life/.

5. Jan P. Piek, Lisa Dawson, Leigh M. Smith, and Natalie Gasson, "The Role of Early Fine and Gross Motor Development on Later Motor and Cognitive Ability," *Human Movement Science* 27, no. 5 (October 2008): 668–681.

6. "CDC's Developmental Milestones," Centers for Disease Control and Prevention, last modified December 29, 2022, https://www.cdc.gov/ncbddd/actearly/milestones/index .html.

7. Hannah Yoo and Dana M. Mihaila, "Rooting Reflex," *StatPearls* (updated April 28, 2022), https://www.ncbi.nlm.nih.gov/books/NBK557636/.

8. Yoo and Mihaila, "Rooting Reflex."

9. Piek et al., "The Role of Early Fine and Gross Motor Development on Later Motor and Cognitive Ability."

10. Raisingchildren.net.

11. "CDC's Developmental Milestones."

12. Yoo and Mihaila, "Rooting Reflex."

13. "CDC's Developmental Milestones."

14. "Babies: Development," raisingchildren.net.au, accessed January 29, 2023, https:// raisingchildren.net.au/babies/development.

15. "CDC's Developmental Milestones"; "Babies: Development."

16. "Important Developmental Milestones: A Timeline for Typical Development," Brain Balance, accessed January 29, 2023, https://www.brainbalancecenters.com/blog/important-developmental-milestones-timeline-typical-development.

17. "CDC's Developmental Milestones"; "Babies: Development."

18. "CDC's Developmental Milestones"; "Babies: Development."

19. "CDC's Developmental Milestones"; "Babies: Development."

20. "Babies: Development."

21. "CDC's Developmental Milestones."

22. "CDC's Developmental Milestones"; "The Growing Child: School Age (6 to 12 years)," Stanford Medicine Children's Health, accessed January 29, 2023, https://www.stanfordchildrens.org/en/topic/default?id=the-growing-child-school-age-6-to-12-years-90-P02278.

23. "The Growing Child: School Age (6 to 12 years)"; "CDC's Developmental Milestones."

24. "The Growing Child: School Age (6 to 12 years)."

25. Julia Brailovskaia, Hans-Werner Bierhoff, Elke Rohmann, Friederike Raeder, and Jürgen Margraf, "The Relationship between Narcissism, Intensity of Facebook Use, Facebook Flow and Facebook Addiction," *Addictive Behavior Reports* 11 (June 2020): 100265, DOI: 10.1016/j.abrep.2020.100265.

26. Matt Richtel, "Children's Screen Time Has Soared in the Pandemic, Alarming Parents and Researchers," *New York Times*, January 16, 2021, https://www.nytimes.com/2021/01/16/health/covid-kids-tech-use.html.

27. Kennon M. Sheldon and Sonja Lyubomirsky, "The Challenge of Staying Happier: Testing the Hedonic Adaptation Prevention Model," *Personality and Social Psychology Bulletin* 38, no. 5 (February 2012): 670–680, DOI: 10.1177/0146167212436400.

Chapter 6

1. Arif Hamid, Jeffrey R. Pettibone, Omar S. Mabrouk, Vaughn L. Hetrick, Robert Schmidt, Caitlin M. Vander Weele, Robert T. Kennedy, et al., "Mesolimbic Dopamine Signals the Value of Work," *Nature Neuroscience* 19 (November 23, 2015): 117–126.

2. "Dopamine Affects How Brain Decides Whether a Goal Is Worth the Effort," National Institutes of Health, March 31, 2020, https://www.nih.gov/news-events/nih-research-matters/dopamine-affects-how-brain-decides-whether-goal-worth-effort.

3. "Reading and Mathematics Scores Decline during Covid-19 Pandemic," Nation's Report Card, accessed January 29, 2023, https://www.nationsreportcard.gov/highlights/ltt/2022/.

4. Doug Howard, "Commentary: Virtual Learning Is Virtually No Education at All," *Baltimore Sun*, August 13, 2020, https://www.baltimoresun.com/maryland/carroll/opinion/cc-op-community-voices-081320-20200813-blvzznuixjahrcoknvicun77re-story.html.

5. Per Engzell, Arun Frey, and Mark D. Verhagen, "Learning Loss Due to School Closures during the COVID-19 Pandemic," *Proceedings of the National Academy of Sciences* 118, no. 17 (April 27, 2021): e2022376118, DOI: 10.1073/pnas.2022376118.

6. Megan Kuhfeld, James Soland, and Karyn Lewis, "Test Score Patterns across Three COVID-19-Impacted School Years," *Educational Researcher* 51, no. 7 (June 30, 2022), https://journals.sagepub.com/doi/10.3102/0013189X221109178.

7. Clea Simon, "How COVID Taught America about Inequity in Education," *Harvard Gazette*, July 9, 2021, https://news.harvard.edu/gazette/story/2021/07/how-covid-taught-america-about-inequity-in-education/.

8. Dana Goldstein, "It's 'Alarming': Children Are Seriously Behind in Reading," *New York Times*, March 8, 2022, https://www.nytimes.com/2022/03/08/us/pandemic-schools-reading-crisis.html.

9. University of Virginia, School of Education and Human Development, "Examining the Impact of COVID-19 on the Identification of At-Risk Students: Fall 2021 Literacy Screening Findings," https://literacy.virginia.edu/sites/g/files/jsddwu1006/files/2022-04/PALS_StateReport_Fall_2021.pdf.

10. Megan Kuhfeld, Jim Soland, Karyn Lewis, and Emily Morton, "The Pandemic Has Had Devastating Impacts on Learning. What Will It Take to Help Students Catch Up?" Brookings Institute, March 3, 2022, https://www.brookings.edu/blog/brown-center-chalkboard/2022/03/03/the-pandemic-has-had-devastating-impacts-on-learning-what-will-it-take-to-help-students-catch-up/.

11. "Medication Doesn't Help Kids with ADHD Learn," Neuroscience News, May 24, 2022, https://neurosciencenews.com/adhd-medication-learning-20647/.

12. Science Daily, "Dyslexics Show a Difference in Sensory Processing," December 21, 2016, https://www.sciencedaily.com/releases/2016/12/161221125517.htm.

13. Martijn P. Van den Heuvel and Olaf Sporns, "Network Hubs in the Human Brain," *Trends in Cognitive Sciences* 17, no. 2 (December 2013): 683–696, https://www.cell.com/trends/cognitive-sciences/fulltext/S1364-6613(13)00216-7#:~:text=Hubs%20are%20central%20in%20brain,susceptible%20to%20disconnection%20and%20dysfunction.

14. "Learning Difficulties Due to Poor Connectivity, Not Specific Brain Regions, Study Shows," University of Cambridge Research (February 27, 2020), https://www.cam.ac.uk/research/news/learning-difficulties-due-to-poor-connectivity-not-specific-brain-regions-study-shows.

15. Roma Siugzdaite, Joe Bathelt, Joni Holmes, and Duncan E. Astle, "Transdiagnostic Brain Mapping in Developmental Disorders," *Current Biology* 30, no. 7 (February 27, 2020): 1245–1257, https://www.cell.com/current-biology/fulltext/S0960-9822(20)30158-5.

16. "Early Brain Development and Health," Centers for Disease Control and Prevention, last modified March 25, 2022, https://www.cdc.gov/ncbddd/childdevelopment/early-brain-development.html.

17. "Ages 0–2," Keep Connected, https://keepconnected.searchinstitute.org/understanding-ages-and-stages/ages-0-2/#:~:text=Infants%20and%20toddlers%20learn%20by,a%20vocabulary%20of%2050%20words.

18. "CDC's Developmental Milestones," Centers for Disease Control and Prevention, last modified December 29, 2022, https://www.cdc.gov/ncbddd/actearly/milestones/index.html.

19. "CDC's Developmental Milestones."

20. "Early Brain Development and Health."

21. Jérémie Blanchette Sarrasin, Lorie-Marlène Brault Foisy, Geneviève Allaire-Duquette, and Steve Masson, "Understanding Your Brain to Help You Learn Better," *Frontiers for Young Minds* 8, no. 54 (May 14, 2020), DOI: 10.3389/frym.2020.00054.

22. Claire Gillespie, "This Is Why We Associate Memories So Strongly with Specific Smells," VeryWellMind, October 4, 2021, https://www.verywellmind.com/why-do-we-associate -memories-so-strongly-with-specific-smells-5203963#:~:text=Scientists%20believe%20 that%20smell%20and,very%20vivid%20when%20it%20happens.

23. Sarrasin et al., "Understanding Your Brain to Help You Learn Better."

24. "CDC's Developmental Milestones"; "Important Developmental Milestones: A Timeline for Typical Development," Brain Balance, accessed January 29, 2023, https://www.brain balancecenters.com/blog/important-developmental-milestones-timeline-typical -development.

25. "Important Developmental Milestones."

26. "Important Developmental Milestones"; "The Growing Child: School Age (6 to 12 years)," Stanford Medicine Children's Health, accessed January 29, 2023, https://www .stanfordchildrens.org/en/topic/default?id=the-growing-child-school-age-6-to-12-years -90-P02278.

27. "The Growing Child: School Age (6 to 12 years)."

28. "The Growing Child: School Age (6 to 12 years)."

29. "The Growing Child: School Age (6 to 12 years)."

30. "The Growing Child: School Age (6 to 12 years)."

31. Noemi Hahn, John J. Foxe, and Sophie Molholm, "Impairments of Multisensory Integration and Cross-Sensory Learning as Pathways to Dyslexia," *Neuroscience and Biobehavioral Reviews* 47 (November 2014): 384–392, DOI: 10.1016/j.neubiorev .2014.09.007.

32. Monica Brady-Myerov, *Listen Wise: Teach Students to Be Better Listeners* (San Francisco: Jossey-Bass, 2022).

33. Julie Beck, "Study: For Memory, Hearing Is Worse than Seeing or Feeling," *The Atlantic* (March 4, 2014), accessed January 23, 2023, https://www.theatlantic.com/health /archive/2014/03/study-for-memory-hearing-is-worse-than-seeing-or-feeling /284184/.

34. Ueli Suter and Rudolf Martini, "Chapter 19: Myelination," in *Peripheral Neuropathy*, 4th ed., edited by Peter J. Dyck and P. K. Thomas (Philadelphia: W.B. Saunders, 2005), 411–431, DOI: 10.1016/B978-0-7216-9491-7.50022-3.

35. "Important Developmental Milestones."

36. "Important Developmental Milestones."

37. "Important Developmental Milestones."

38. Amanda Morin, "Developmental Milestones for High-Schoolers," Understood, accessed January 29, 2023, https://www.understood.org/en/articles/developmental-milestones -for-typical-high-schoolers; "Understanding Your Pre-Teen," raisingchildren.net.au, accessed January 29, 2023, https://raisingchildren.net.au/pre-teens/development /understanding-your-pre-teen/brain-development-teens#:~:text=Adolescence%20is %20a%20time%20of,time%2C%20other%20connections%20are%20strengthened.

Chapter 7

1. Erin Einhorn, "One Classroom but Very Different Students: Why It's Now Harder for Children to Catch Up in School," NBC News, July 19, 2022, https://www.nbcnews .com/news/us-news/student-test-scores-pandemic-rcna38106.

2. Jill Seladi-Schulman, "What Is the Vagus Nerve?" VeryWellHealth, last modified July 22, 2022, https://www.healthline.com/human-body-maps/vagus-nerve.

3. Elizabeth Dougherty, "Anger Management," *Harvard Medicine*, Autumn 2022, accessed January 29, 2023, https://hms.harvard.edu/magazine/science-emotion/anger -management.

4. M. T. Birnie and T. Z. Baram, "Principles of Emotional Brain Circuit Maturation," *Science* 376, no. 6597 (June 3, 2022): 1055–1056, DOI: 10.1126/science.abn4016.

5. "It's Never Too Early to Get Your Baby on the Right Pathway," Pathways, https:// pathways.org/baby-on-the-way/#:~:text=If%20you're%20using%20the,can%20be %20found%2C%20the%20better.

6. "Important Developmental Milestones: A Timeline for Typical Development," Brain Balance, accessed January 29, 2023, https://www.brainbalancecenters.com/blog /important-developmental-milestones-timeline-typical-development.

7. "Important Developmental Milestones."

8. "Important Developmental Milestones."

9. "Important Developmental Milestones."

10. "Important Developmental Milestones."

11. Jay L. Hoecker, "I've Heard a Lot about the Terrible Twos. Why Are 2-Year Olds so Difficult?" Mayo Clinic, February 23, 2022, https://www.mayoclinic.org/healthy -lifestyle/infant-and-toddler-health/expert-answers/terrible-twos/faq-20058314.

12. Summarized in Donna Christiano, "What to Expect from the Terrible Twos," HealthLine, February 25, 2019, https://www.healthline.com/health/parenting/terrible -twos#:~:text=Signs%20to%20look%20for%20include,to%2020%20times%20a %20day. The original study was Heidelise Als et al., "A Three-Center, Randomized, Controlled Trial of Individualized Developmental Care for Very Low Birth Weight Preterm Infants: Medical, Neurodevelopmental, Parenting, and Caregiving Effects," *Journal of Developmental and Behavioral Pediatrics* 24, no. 6 (December 2003): 399–408.

13. Christiano, "What to Expect from the Terrible Twos."

14. "The Growing Child: School Age (6 to 12 years)," Stanford Medicine Children's Health, accessed January 29, 2023, https://www.stanfordchildrens.org/en/topic/default?id=the -growing-child-school-age-6-to-12-years-90-P02278.

15. "Important Developmental Milestones."

16. "Important Developmental Milestones."

17. "Developmental Milestones," C. S. Mott Children's Hospital, last modified January 2022, https://www.mottchildren.org/posts/your-child/developmental-milestones.

18. "Important Developmental Milestones."

19. "Important Developmental Milestones."

20. "Important Developmental Milestones."

21. Torben Ott, Paul Masset, and Adam Kepecs, "The Neurobiology of Confidence: From Beliefs to Neurons," *Cold Spring Harbor Symposia on Quantitative Biology* 83 (2018): 9–16, DOI: 10.1101/sqb.2018.83.038794.

22. "Important Developmental Milestones."

23. "Important Developmental Milestones."

24. Adele Diamond, "Activities and Programs That Improve Children's Executive Functions," *Current Directions in Psychological Science* 21, no. 5 (October 2012): 335–341, DOI: 10.1177/0963721412453722.
25. Weiyan Yin, Tengfei Li, Peter J. Mucha, Jessica R. Cohen, Hongtu Zhu, Ziliang Li, and Weili Lin, "Altered Neural Flexibility in Children with Attention-Deficit/Hyperactivity Disorder," *Molecular Psychiatry* 27 (July 22, 2022): 4673–4679.
26. Diamond, "Activities and Programs That Improve Children's Executive Functions."
27. Bruno Bonaz, Valérie Sinniger, and Sonia Pellissier, "The Vagus Nerve in the Neuro-Immune Axis: Implications in the Pathology of the Gastrointestinal Tract," *Frontiers in Immunology* 8 (November 2, 2017): 1–14, DOI: 10.3389/fimmu.2017.01452.

Chapter 8

1. "Data and Statistics on Children's Mental Health," Centers for Disease Control and Prevention, last modified June 3, 2022, https://www.cdc.gov/childrensmentalhealth /data.html#:~:text=Depression%20and%20anxiety%20have%20increased,8.4%25%20 in%202011%E2%80%932012.&text=%E2%80%9CEver%20having%20been %20diagnosed%20with%20anxiety%E2%80%9D%20increased%20from%205.5 %25,6.4%25%20in%202011%E2%80%932012.
2. Damian F. Santomauro, Ana M. Mantilla Herrera, Jamileh Shadid, Peng Zheng, Charlie Ashbaugh, David M. Pigott, Cristiana Abbafati, Christopher Adolph, et al., "Global Prevalence and Burden of Depressive and Anxiety Disorders in 204 Countries and Territories in 2020 Due to the COVID-19 Pandemic," *The Lancet* 398, no. 10312 (November 6, 2021): 1700–1712, https://www.thelancet.com/journals/lancet/article /PIIS0140-6736(21)02143-7/fulltext.
3. From Google Search, "Anxiety," https://www.google.com/search?q=definition+of+ anxiety&rlz=1C1GEWG_enUS1004US1004&oq=definition+of+anxiety&aqs=chrome .69i57j0i512l9.4367j0j4&sourceid=chrome&ie=UTF-8.
4. American Psychological Association, "APA Dictionary of Psychology—Anxiety," accessed March 15, 2023, https://dictionary.apa.org/anxiety.
5. Kaitlin Vogel, "When Anxiety Manifests in Anger," PsychCentral, March 28, 2022, https://psychcentral.com/anxiety/anxiety-and-anger.
6. Sigrid Breit, Aleksandra Kupferberg, Gerhard Rogler, and Gregor Hasler, "Vagus Nerve as Modulator of the Brain–Gut Axis in Psychiatric and Inflammatory Disorders," *Frontiers in Psychiatry* 9 (March 13, 2018), DOI: 10.3389/fpsyt.2018.00044.
7. "Understanding the Stress Response," Harvard Medical School, July 6, 2020, https:// www.health.harvard.edu/staying-healthy/understanding-the-stress-response#:~:text =It%20triggers%20the%20fight%2Dor,after%20the%20danger%20has%20passed.
8. "What Is a Cortisol Test?" WebMD, December 13, 2022, https://www.webmd.com /a-to-z-guides/what-is-cortisol.
9. Bruce S. McEwen and John H. Morrison, "The Brain on Stress: Vulnerability and Plasticity of the Prefrontal Cortex over the Life Course," *Neuron* 79, no. 1 (July 10, 2013): 16–29, DOI: 10.1016/j.neuron.2013.06.028.
10. Xin Zhang, Tong Ge, Guanghao Yin, Ranji Cui, Guoqing Zhao, and Wei Yang, "Stress-Induced Functional Alterations in Amygdala: Implications for Neuropsychiatric

Diseases," *Frontiers in Neuroscience* 12, no. 367 (May 29, 2018), DOI: 10.3389/fnins .2018.00367.

11. Breit et al., "Vagus Nerve as Modulator of the Brain–Gut Axis in Psychiatric and Inflammatory Disorders."

12. "How to Reduce Cortisol and Turn Down the Dial on Stress," Cleveland Clinic, August 27, 2020, https://health.clevelandclinic.org/how-to-reduce-cortisol-and-turn -down-the-dial-on-stress/.

13. Christopher André, "Proper Breathing Brings Better Health," *Scientific American*, January 15, 2019, https://www.scientificamerican.com/article/proper-breathing-brings -better-health/.

14. Karen Young, "Fear and Anxiety—An Age by Age Guide to Common Fears, the Reasons for Each and How to Manage Them," HeySigmund, accessed January 29, 2023, https:// www.heysigmund.com/age-by-age-guide-to-fears/.

15. Young, "Fear and Anxiety—An Age by Age Guide to Common Fears, the Reasons for Each and How to Manage Them."

16. Young, "Fear and Anxiety—An Age by Age Guide to Common Fears, the Reasons for Each and How to Manage Them."

17. Young, "Fear and Anxiety—An Age by Age Guide to Common Fears, the Reasons for Each and How to Manage Them."

18. Young, "Fear and Anxiety—An Age by Age Guide to Common Fears, the Reasons for Each and How to Manage Them."

19. Young, "Fear and Anxiety—An Age by Age Guide to Common Fears, the Reasons for Each and How to Manage Them."

20. Valentin Magnon, Frédéric Dutheil, and Guillaume T. Vallet, "Benefits from One Session of Deep and Slow Breathing on Vagal Tone and Anxiety in Young and Older Adults," *Scientific Reports* 11 (September 29, 2021), DOI: 10.1038/s41598-021 -98736-9.

21. Young, "Fear and Anxiety—An Age by Age Guide to Common Fears, the Reasons for Each and How to Manage Them."

22. "Exercising to Relax," Harvard Medical School, July 7, 2020, https://www.health .harvard.edu/staying-healthy/exercising-to-relax.

23. Pragati Rokade, "Release of Endomorphin Hormone and Its Effects on Our Body and Moods: A Review," *International Conference on Chemical, Biological and Environment Sciences* 431127, no. 215 (2011/2012): 436 438.

24. Emma E. A. Cohen, Robin Ejsmond-Frey, Nicola Knight, and R. I. M. Dunbar, "Rowers' High: Behavioural Synchrony Is Correlated with Elevated Pain Thresholds," *Biology Letters* 6, no. 1 (February 23, 2010):106–108, DOI: 10.1098/rsbl.2009.0670.

25. Bethany E. Kok, Kimberly A. Coffey, Michael A. Cohn, Lahnna I. Catalino, Tanya Vacharkulksemsuk, Sara B. Algoe, Mary Brantley, and Barbara L. Fredrickson, "How Positive Emotions Build Physical Health: Perceived Positive Social Connections Account for the Upward Spiral between Positive Emotions and Vagal Tone," *Psychological Science* 24, no. 7 (July 1, 2013): 1123–1132, DOI: 10.1177/0956797612470827.

26. B. Bonaz, T. Bazin, and S. Pellissier, "The Vagus Nerve at the Interface of the Microbiota-Gut-Brain Axis," *Frontiers in Neuroscience* 12 (February 7, 2018): 49, DOI: 10.3389/fnins.2018.00049.

Chapter 9

1. Associated Press, "Seattle's Schools Are Suing Tech Giants for Harming Young People's Mental Health," National Public Radio, January 8, 2023, https://www.npr.org/2023 /01/08/1147735477/seattles-schools-are-suing-tech-giants-for-harming-young-peoples -mental-health#:~:text=on%20mobile%20devices.-,On%20Friday%2C%20Jan.%20 6%2C%202023%2C%20Seattle%20Public%20Schools,mental%20health%20crisis %20among%20youth.

2. Clare Timbie and Helen Barbas, "Pathways for Emotions: Specializations in the Amygdalar, Mediodorsal Thalamic, and Posterior Orbitofrontal Network," *Journal of Neuroscience* 35, no. 34 (August 26, 2015): 11976–11987, DOI: 10.1523/JNEUROSCI .2157-15.2015.

3. Joanna Moncrieff, Ruth E. Cooper, Tom Stockmann, Simone Amendola, Michael P. Hengartner, and Mark Horowitz, "The Serotonin Theory of Depression: A Systematic Umbrella Review of the Evidence," *Molecular Psychiatry* (July 20, 2022), DOI: 10.1038 /s41380-022-01661-0.

4. Thomas Insel, "Towards a New Understanding of Mental Illness," filmed April 16, 2013, TED video, 13:03, https://www.youtube.com/watch?v=PeZ-U0pj9LI.

5. "Sleep in Middle and High School Students," Centers for Disease Control and Prevention, last modified September 10, 2020, https://www.cdc.gov/healthyschools /features/students-sleep.htm#:~:text=The%20American%20Academy%20of%20Sleep ,10%20hours%20per%2024%20hours.

6. Joshua L. Hudson, Jamie I. Baum, Eva C. Diaz, and Elisabet Børsheim, "Dietary Protein Requirements in Children: Methods for Consideration," *Nutrients* 13, no. 5 (May 5, 2021): 1554, DOI: 10.3390/nu13051554.

7. Stephanie Pappas, "What Do We Really Know about Kids and Screens?" *Monitor on Psychology* 3, no. 51 (June 30, 2022), https://www.apa.org/monitor/2020/04/cover -kids-screens#:~:text=AAP%20calls%20for%20no%20screen,of%20screen%20time %20per%20day.

8. "How Many Hours in a Lifetime Do We Sleep?" Healthy Journal, https://www.the healthyjournal.com/frequently-asked-questions/how-many-hours-in-a-lifetime-do -we-sleep.

9. Ferris Jabr, "Why Your Brain Needs More Dopamine," *Scientific American*, October 5, 2013, https://www.scientificamerican.com/article/mental-downtime/#:~:text =Downtime%20replenishes%20the%20brain%27s%20stores,stable%20memories %20in%20everyday%20life.

10. Simon Makin, "Deep Sleep Gives Your Brain a Deep Clean," *Scientific American*, November 1, 2019, https://www.scientificamerican.com/article/deep-sleep-gives-your -brain-a-deep-clean1/.

11. "Sleep, Learning, and Memory," Harvard Medical School, last modified December 18, 2007, https://healthysleep.med.harvard.edu/healthy/matters/benefits-of-sleep /learning-memory.

12. "Sleep, Learning, and Memory."

13. Jillian Kubala, "Essential Amino Acids: Definition, Benefits, and Food Sources," HealthLine, February 3, 2022, https://www.healthline.com/nutrition/essential-amino

-acids#:~:text=Amino%20acids%2C%20often%20referred%20to,meat%2C%20fish
%2C%20and%20soybeans.

14. Kubala, "Essential Amino Acids: Definition, Benefits, and Food Sources."

15. Charlotte Lillis, "What Are Some Slow-Release Carbs?" MedicalNewsToday, June 27, 2019, https://www.medicalnewstoday.com/articles/325586.

16. Lillis, "What Are Some Slow-Release Carbs?"

17. Evan Forth, Benjamin Buehner, Ana Storer, Cassandra Sgarbossa, Roumen Milev, and Arthi Chinna Meyyappan, "Systematic Review of Probiotics as an Adjuvant Treatment for Psychiatric Disorders," *Frontiers of Behavioral Neuroscience* 17 (February 9, 2023): 1–10, https://www.frontiersin.org/articles/10.3389/fnbeh.2023.1111349/full.

18. Johns Hopkins Medicine, "The Brain-Gut Connection," https://www.hopkinsmedicine .org/health/wellness-and-prevention/the-brain-gut-connection, accessed March 15, 2023.

19. Lu Liu and Gang Zhu, "Gut-Brain Axis and Mood Disorder," *Frontiers of Psychiatry* 9 (May 29, 2018): 1–8, DOI: 10.3389/fpsyt.2018.00223.

20. Carl W. Cotman and Nicole C. Berchtold, "Exercise: A Behavioral Intervention to Enhance Brain Health and Plasticity," *Trends in Neuroscience* 6, no. 25 (June 2002): 295–301, DOI: 10.1016/s0166-2236(02)02143-4.

21. Kelly McGonigal, "Five Surprising Ways Exercise Changes Your Brain," *Greater Good Magazine*, January 6, 2020, https://greatergood.berkeley.edu/article/item/five _surprising_ways_exercise_changes_your_brain#:~:text=Exercise%20can%20make%20 your%20brain%20more%20sensitive%20to%20joy&text=Over%20time%2C%20 regular%20exercise%20remodels,expand%20your%20capacity%20for%20joy.

22. Sean Myers, "Study Shows Majority of Children under Five Are Getting Too Much Screen Time," University of Calgary, February 14, 2022, https://arts.ucalgary.ca/news /node/30114#:~:text=A%20large%20new%20University%20of,of%20one%20hour %20per%20day.

23. "Sleep in Middle and High School Students."

24. Hudson et al., "Dietary Protein Requirements in Children: Methods for Consideration."

25. Pappas, "What Do We Really Know about Kids and Screens?"

26. Glenn R. Fox, Jonas Kaplan, Hanna Damasio, and Antonio Damasio, "Neural Correlates of Gratitude," *Frontiers in Psychology* 6 (September 30, 2015), DOI: 10.3389 /fpsyg.2015.01491.

27. Flow Research Collective, "Flow, Emotional Intelligence, Mindfulness and the Brain with a Legend in the Field," May 3, 2021, https://www.flowresearchcollective.com /radio/40.

28. Linda Roszak Burton, "The Neuroscience of Gratitude," Wharton Health Care, accessed January 29, 2023, https://www.whartonhealthcare.org/the_neuroscience_of_gratitude.

29. Wikipedia, "Mindfulness," accessed March 15, 2023, https://en.wikipedia.org/wiki /Mindfulness.

30. "Sleep in Middle and High School Students."

31. Hudson et al., "Dietary Protein Requirements in Children: Methods for Consideration."

32. "Screen Time by Age Guide," Brain Balance Centers, accessed January 29, 2023, https:// www.brainbalancecenters.com/blog/screen-time-by-age-guide.

33. The American Academy for Pediatrics has historically recommended no more than two hours a day of screen time, but they have recently updated their guidance to reflect that the technology is interwoven in our daily lives now. The recommendations have added guidelines such as no technology at mealtimes or an hour before bed. They also want to ensure at least sixty minutes a day of physical activity. According to the American Academy of Child and Adolescent Psychiatry, usage of technology by teens is up to nine hours per day using a combination of smartphone, tablet, TV, gaming console, and computer. See Amy Morin, "How Much Should You Limit Kids' Screen Time and Electronics Use?" VeryWellFamily, last modified March 6, 2021, https://www.very wellfamily.com/american-academy-pediatrics-screen-time-guidelines-1094883; "Resource Centers," American Academy of Child and Adolescent Psychiatry, accessed January 29, 2023, http://www.AACAP.org.

34. Flow Research Collective, "The Dangers of Having a Passion and a Purpose," May 20, 2021, https://www.flowresearchcollective.com/radio/42.

35. Shiv Sudhakar, "Why Most New Year's Resolutions Fail—A New Approach to Consider," *New York Post*, December 31, 2022, https://nypost.com/2022/12/31/why -most-new-years-resolutions-fail-and-a-new-approach-to-consider/.

36. "Good Social Relationships Are the Most Consistent Predictor of a Happy Life," Stanford Medicine, October 18, 2019, http://ccare.stanford.edu/press_posts/good -social-relationships-are-the-most-consistent-predictor-of-a-happy-life.

INDEX